Practical Case Studies in Hypertension Management

Series editor
Giuliano Tocci
Rome, Italy

The aim of the book series "Practical Case Studies in Hypertension Management" is to provide physicians who treat hypertensive patients having different cardiovascular risk profiles with an easy-to-access tool that will enhance their clinical practice, improve average blood pressure control, and reduce the incidence of major hypertension-related complications. To achieve these ambitious goals, each volume presents and discusses a set of paradigmatic clinical cases relating to different scenarios in hypertension. These cases will serve as a basis for analyzing best practice and highlight problems in implementing the recommendations contained in international guidelines regarding diagnosis and treatment. While the available guidelines have contributed significantly in improving the diagnostic process, cardiovascular risk stratification, and therapeutic management in patients with essential hypertension, they are of relatively limited help to physicians in daily clinical practice when approaching individual patients with hypertension, and this is particularly true when choosing among different drug classes and molecules. By discussing exemplary clinical cases that may better represent clinical practice in a "real world" setting, this series will assist physicians in selecting the best diagnostic and therapeutic options.

More information about this series at http://www.springer.com/series/13624

Giuliano Tocci

Hypertension and Organ Damage

A Case-Based Guide to Management

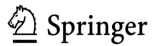 Springer

Giuliano Tocci
Department of Clinical and Molecular Medicine
University of Rome Sapienza St Andrea Hospital
Rome
Italy

ISSN 2364-6632   ISSN 2364-6640 (electronic)
Practical Case Studies in Hypertension Management
ISBN 978-3-319-25095-3   ISBN 978-3-319-25097-7 (eBook)
DOI 10.1007/978-3-319-25097-7

Library of Congress Control Number: 2015958250

Springer Cham Heidelberg New York Dordrecht London

Printed on acid-free paper

Springer International Publishing AG Switzerland is part of Springer Science+Business Media (www.springer.com)

Preface

The natural history of hypertension is characterised by the development and progression of structural and functional abnormalities at cardiac, vascular and renal levels, which are in turn related to an increased risk of developing major cardiovascular, cerebrovascular and renal complications.

During this course, the proper assessment and prompt regression of hypertension-related organ damage represent fundamental steps for the clinical management of hypertension. In fact, effective blood pressure control under specific antihypertensive drug therapies can interfere with the progression and promote the regression of markers of organ damage, being associated with improved prognosis and reduced risk of complications. In particular, the identification of serial changes of different signs of organ damage has been viewed by physicians as an easy, simple and cost-effectiveness way to evaluate the individual global cardiovascular risk profile and to test the effectiveness of antihypertensive strategy in patients with hypertension at high cardiovascular risk.

In this first volume of the series *Practical Case Studies in Hypertension Management*, the clinical management of paradigmatic cases of patients with hypertension and different markers of organ damage will be discussed, focusing on the different diagnostic criteria currently available for identifying the presence or the absence of these markers as well as on the different therapeutic options now recommended for reducing progression and promoting regression of hypertension-related signs of organ damage.

Rome, Italy   Giuliano Tocci

Contents

Clinical Case 1
Patient with Essential Hypertension and Left Ventricular Hypertrophy

1.1 Clinical Case Presentation

A 54-year-old, Caucasian male, gardener, presented to the outpatient clinic for recently uncontrolled hypertension.

He has history of essential hypertension by more than 15 years, initially treated with a combination therapy based on beta-blocker (atenolol 100 mg) and diuretic (chlorthalidone 25 mg).

About 10 years ago, for incoming asthenia and sexual disturbances, he was moved to a combination therapy based on angiotensin-converting enzyme (ACE) inhibitor (ramipril 10 mg) and thiazide diuretic (hydrochlorothiazide 25 mg), with satisfactory BP control at home and no relevant side effects or adverse reactions.

By about 6 months, he reported uncontrolled blood pressure (BP) levels measured at home and effort dyspnoea. He also described inconstant cough. For these reasons, his referring physician prescribed furosemide 25 mg daily in addition to current pharmacological therapy, albeit with limited improvement on BP control.

G. Tocci, *Hypertension and Organ Damage: A Case-Based Guide to Management*, Practical Case Studies in Hypertension Management, DOI 10.1007/978-3-319-25097-7_1,
© Springer International Publishing Switzerland 2016

Family History

He has paternal history of hypertension and stroke and maternal history of diabetes and hypercholesterolemia. He also has one sibling with hypertension.

Clinical History

He was previous smoker (about 10–20 cigarettes daily) for more than 20 years until the age of 45 years. He also has two additional modifiable cardiovascular risk factors, including sedentary life habits and overweight (visceral obesity). There are no further cardiovascular risk factors, associated clinical conditions or non-cardiovascular diseases.

Physical Examination

- Weight: 88 kg
- Height: 174 cm
- Body mass index (BMI): 29.1 kg/m^2
- Waist circumference: 118 cm
- Respiration: normal
- Heart sounds: S1–S2 regular, normal and no murmurs
- Resting pulse: regular rhythm with normal heart rate (67 beats/min)
- Carotid arteries: no murmurs
- Femoral and foot arteries: palpable

Haematological Profile

- Haemoglobin: 15.1 g/dL
- Haematocrit: 49.3 %
- Fasting plasma glucose: 87 mg/dL

- Fasting lipids: total cholesterol (TOT-C): 174 mg/dl; low-density lipoprotein cholesterol (LDL-C): 111 mg/dl; high-density lipoprotein cholesterol (HDL-C): 39 mg/dl; triglycerides (TG) 122 mg/dl
- Electrolytes: sodium, 146 mEq/L; potassium, 4.2 mEq/L
- Serum uric acid: 4.1 mg/dL
- Renal function: urea 24 mg/dl, creatinine, 0.8 mg/dL; creatinine clearance (Cockcroft–Gault): 130 ml/min; estimated glomerular filtration rate (eGFR) (MDRD): 110 mL/min/1.73 m²
- Urine analysis (dipstick): normal
- Albuminuria: 12.2 mg/24 h
- Normal liver function tests
- Normal thyroid function tests

Blood Pressure Profile

- Home BP (average): 160–165/100 mmHg
- Sitting BP: 164/106 mmHg (right arm); 166/107 mmHg (left arm)
- Standing BP: 167/108 mmHg at 1 min
- 24-h BP: 161/112 mmHg; HR: 67 bpm
- Daytime BP: 162/113 mmHg; HR: 71 bpm
- Night-time BP: 154/103 mmHg; HR: 61 bpm

A 24-h ambulatory blood pressure profile is illustrated in Fig. 1.1.

12-Lead Electrocardiogram

Sinus rhythm with normal heart rate (63 bpm), normal atrioventricular and intraventricular conduction and ST-segment abnormalities without signs of LVH (aVL 0.7 mV, Sokolow–Lyon 2.1 mV, Cornell voltage 1.4 mV, Cornell product 130 mV*ms) (Fig. 1.2).

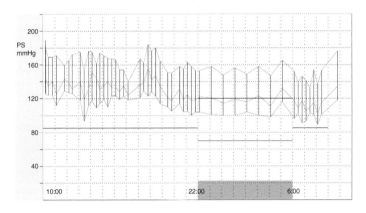

FIGURE 1.1 24-h ambulatory blood pressure profile at first visit

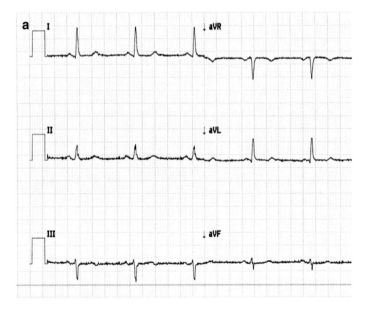

FIGURE 1.2 (**a**, **b**) Sinus rhythm with normal heart rate (63 bpm), normal atrioventricular and intraventricular conduction and ST-segment abnormalities without signs of LVH

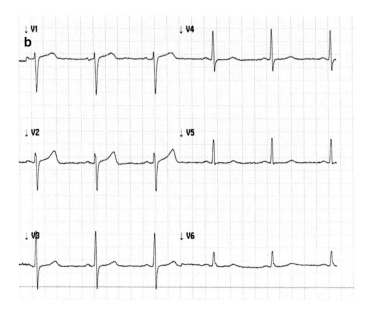

FIGURE 1.2 (continued)

Vascular Ultrasound

Carotid: Intima–media thickness at both carotid levels (right, 1.0 mm, Fig. 1.3a; left, 0.9 mm, Fig. 1.3b) without evidence of atherosclerotic plaques.

Renal: Intima–media thickness at both renal arteries without evidence of atherosclerotic plaques. Normal Doppler examination at both right and left arteries. Normal dimension and structure of the abdominal aorta.

Current Treatment

Ramipril 10 mg h 8:00, hydrochlorothiazide 25 mg h 8:00 and furosemide 25 mg h 12:00.

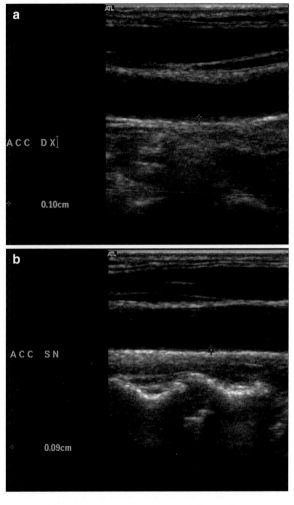

FIGURE 1.3 Intima–media thickness at both carotid levels (right, 1.0 mm (**a**); left, 0.9 mm (**b**), without evidence of atherosclerotic plaques

Diagnosis

Essential (stage 2) hypertension with unsatisfactory BP control on combination therapy. Additional modifiable cardiovascular risk factors (sedentary habits and visceral obesity). No evidence of hypertension-related organ damage nor associated clinical conditions.

> **Which is the global cardiovascular risk profile in this patient?**
>
> Possible answers are:
>
> 1. Low
> 2. Medium
> 3. High
> 4. Very high

Global Cardiovascular Risk Stratification

According to 2013 ESH/ESC global cardiovascular risk stratification [1], this patient has moderate to high cardiovascular risk.

> **Which is the best therapeutic option in this patient?**
> Possible answers are:
>
> 1. Add another drug class (e.g. dihydropyridinic calcium-antagonist).
> 2. Add another drug class (e.g. beta-blocker).
> 3. Add another drug class (e.g. alpha-blocker).
> 4. Switch from ACE inhibitor to angiotensin receptor blocker combined with thiazide diuretic.
> 5. Switch from ACE inhibitor to direct renin inhibitor combined with thiazide diuretic.

Treatment Evaluation

- Stop ACE inhibitor ramipril 10 mg and furosemide 25 mg.
- Start fixed combination therapy with losartan/hydrochlorothiazide 100/25 mg h 8:00.

Prescriptions

- Periodical BP evaluation at home according to recommendations from guidelines
- Regular physical activity and low caloric intake
- Echocardiogram aimed at evaluating left ventricular (LV) mass and function (systolic and diastolic properties)

1.2   Follow-Up (Visit 1) at 6 Weeks

At follow-up visit the patient is in good clinical condition. He started moderate physical activity two times per week with beneficial effects (weight loss and relatively good exercise tolerance). He also reported good adherence to prescribed medications without adverse reactions or drug-related side effects (absence of cough and improved dyspnoea).

Physical Examination

- Weight: 86 kg
- BMI: 28.1 kg/m^2
- Waist circumference: 114 cm
- Resting pulse: regular rhythm with normal heart rate (65 beats/min)
- Other clinical parameters substantially unchanged

Blood Pressure Profile

- Home BP (average): 155/90 mmHg (early morning)
- Sitting BP: 158/92 mmHg (left arm)
- Standing BP: 158/94 mmHg at 1 min

Current Treatment

Losartan/hydrochlorothiazide 100/25 mg h 8:00.

Echocardiogram

Concentric LV hypertrophy (LV mass indexed 128 g/m^2, relative wall thickness 0.53) with normal chamber dimension (LV end-diastolic diameter 49 mm) (Fig. 1.4a), impaired LV relaxation (E/A ratio <1) at both conventional (Fig. 1.4b) and tissue (Fig. 1.4c) Doppler evaluations and normal ejection fraction (LV ejection fraction 66 %, LV fractional shortening 37 %). Normal dimension of aortic root and left atrium. Right ventricle with normal dimension and function. Pericardium without relevant abnormalities.

Mitral (++) and tricuspid (+) regurgitations at Doppler ultrasound examination.

Diagnosis

Essential (stage 2) hypertension with improved BP control on combination therapy without achieving the recommended BP targets. Cardiac organ damage (concentric LV hypertrophy) and impaired LV relaxation. Additional cardiovascular risk factors (visceral obesity).

Which is the global cardiovascular risk profile in this patient?

Possible answers are:

1. Low
2. Medium
3. High
4. Very high

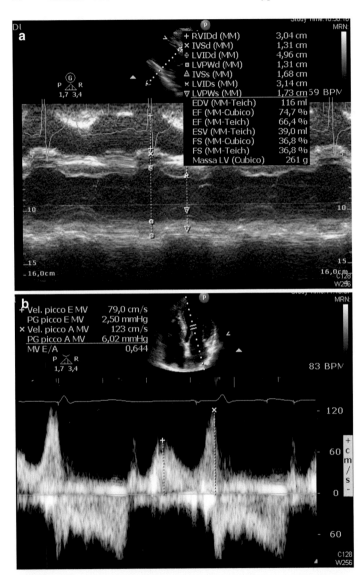

FIGURE 1.4 Echocardiogram at follow-up visit after 6 weeks. Concentric LV hypertrophy with normal chamber dimension (**a**), impaired LV relaxation at both conventional (**b**) and tissue (**c**)

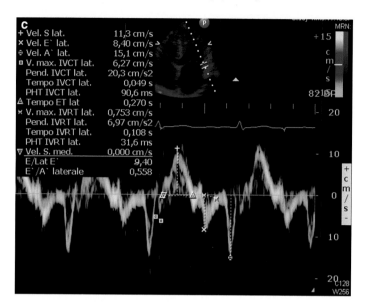

FIGURE 1.4 (continued)

Global Cardiovascular Risk Stratification

The echocardiographic evidence of cardiac organ damage (concentric LV hypertrophy) is able to modify the individual global cardiovascular risk profile. On the basis of the echocardiographic assessment, this patient has moved from moderate to high cardiovascular risk, according to 2013 ESH/ESC global cardiovascular risk stratification [1]. This would lead to an increased 10-year risk of developing cardiovascular disease (morbidity and mortality).

Which is the best therapeutic option in this patient?

Possible answers are:

1. Add another drug class (e.g. dihydropyridinic calcium-antagonist).
2. Add another drug class (e.g. beta-blocker).

(continued)

3. Add another drug class (e.g. alpha-blocker).
4. Switch from angiotensin receptor blocker to direct renin inhibitor combined with thiazide diuretic.

Treatment Evaluation

- Start amlodipine 5 mg h 20:00.
- Maintain losartan/hydrochlorothiazide 100/25 mg h 8:00.

Prescriptions

- Periodical BP evaluation at home according to recommendations from current guidelines.
- Regular physical activity and low caloric intake.

1.3   Follow-Up (Visit 2) at 3 Months

At follow-up visit the patient is in good clinical condition. He maintained regular physical activity two to three times per week with benefits (further weight loss and good exercise tolerance). He also reported good adherence to prescribed medications without adverse reactions or drug-related side effects (absence of dyspnoea).

Physical Examination

- Weight: 83 kg
- BMI: 27.0 kg/m^2
- Waist circumference: 110 cm
- Resting pulse: regular rhythm with 63 beats/min
- Other parameters substantially unchanged

Blood Pressure Profile

- Home BP (average): 145/85 mmHg (early morning)
- Sitting BP: 148/87 mmHg (left arm)
- Standing BP: 148/88 mmHg at 1 min

Current Treatment

Losartan/hydrochlorothiazide 100/25 mg h 8:00; amlodipine 5 mg h 20:00.

Which is the best therapeutic option in this patient?
Possible answers are:

1. Add another drug class (e.g. beta-blocker).
2. Add another drug class (e.g. alpha-blocker).
3. Titrate the dosage of current therapy.
4. Switch from ARB to direct renin inhibitor combined with thiazide diuretic.

Treatment Evaluation

- Titrate the dosage of amlodipine from 5 mg to 10 mg h 20:00.
- Maintain losartan/hydrochlorothiazide 100/25 mg h 8:00.

Prescriptions

- Periodical BP evaluation at home according to recommendations from current guidelines.
- Repeat 12-lead electrocardiogram.
- Repeat 24-h ambulatory BP monitoring to test sustained and effective antihypertensive efficacy of prescribed medications.

1.4   Follow-Up (Visit 2) at 1 Year

At follow-up visit the patient is in good clinical condition. He also reported good adherence to prescribed medications with no adverse reactions or relevant drug-related side effects.

Physical Examination

- Weight: 81 kg
- Body mass index (BMI): 26.7 kg/m^2
- Waist circumference: 110 cm
- Resting pulse: regular rhythm with 65 beats/min
- Other parameters substantially unchanged

Blood Pressure Profile

- Home BP (average): 130/80 mmHg
- Sitting BP: 136/82 mmHg (left arm)
- Standing BP: 138/88 mmHg at 1 min
- 24-h BP: 132/77 mmHg; HR: 78 bpm
- Daytime BP: 134/79 mmHg; HR: 80 bpm
- Night-time BP: 118/66 mmHg; HR: 64 bpm

A 24-h ambulatory blood pressure profile is illustrated in Fig. 1.5.

12-Lead Electrocardiogram

Sinus rhythm with normal heart rate (64 bpm), normal atrio-ventricular and intraventricular conduction and no ST-segment abnormalities or signs of LVH without signs of LVH (aVL 0.8 mV, Sokolow–Lyon 2.7 mV, Cornell voltage 1.8 mV, Cornell product 151 mV*ms) (Fig. 1.6).

Current Treatment

Losartan/hydrochlorothiazide 100/25 mg h 8:00; amlodipine 10 mg h 20:00.

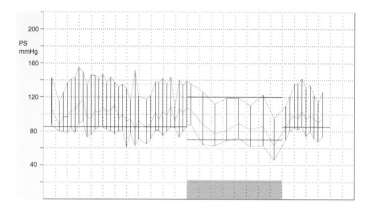

FIGURE 1.5 24-h ambulatory blood pressure profile at follow-up visit after 1 year

Treatment Evaluation

• No changes for current pharmacological therapy

Prescriptions

• Periodical BP evaluation at home according to recommendations from current guidelines
• Regular physical activity and low caloric intake

Which is the most useful diagnostic test to repeat during the follow-up in this patient?

Possible answers are:

1. Electrocardiogram
2. Echocardiogram
3. Vascular Doppler ultrasound
4. Evaluation of renal parameters (e.g. creatininemia, eGFR, ClCr, UACR)
5. 24-h ambulatory BP monitoring

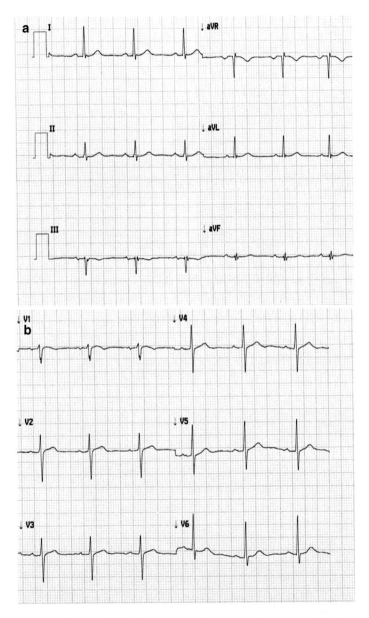

FIGURE 1.6 (**a**, **b**) 12-lead electrocardiogram at follow-up visit after 1 year

1.5 Discussion

Arterial hypertension has been associated to development and progression of cardiac organ damage, namely LV hypertrophy, which in turn is related to an increased risk of coronary events, myocardial infarction, ischemic stroke and congestive heart failure. For these reasons, systematic assessment of LV hypertrophy in all hypertensive patients has been recently reaffirmed and promoted by 2013 European Society of Hypertension (ESH)/European Society of Cardiology (ESC) guidelines on the clinical management of hypertension [1], in order to properly identify and treat those hypertensive patients at high cardiovascular risk.

In this view, the presence of LV hypertrophy can be assessed with various diagnostic tests, although with different levels of sensitivity and specificity and different costs. In a setting clinical practice, the most commonly used tools are represented by conventional 12-lead electrocardiogram and echocardiogram [2–4]. For these tests, specific diagnostic criteria for LV hypertrophy are available, so that physicians can easily assess the presence or absence of cardiac organ damage at first evaluation or during the follow-up of patients with hypertension. For example, several diagnostic criteria are available for electrocardiographic assessment of LV hypertrophy (Table 1.1). The major limitation of electrocardiogram, however, is the high sensitivity and relatively low specificity to detect LV hypertrophy [5, 6]. To overcome this intrinsic limitation, echocardiographic evaluation of LV geometry and function can be assessed. With this examination, the presence of cardiac organ damage can be assessed according to specific diagnostic criteria (Table 1.2).

In this clinical case some aspects deserve a comment. First of all, electrocardiographic evaluation of cardiac organ damage should be always performed at first clinical assessment in all hypertensive patients, in order to evaluate heart rate and rhythm and presence of LV hypertrophy. The search for cardiac organ damage can be further integrated by conventional

TABLE 1.1 Electrocardiographic criteria for the diagnosis of LV hypertrophy

A. Diagnostic criteria recommended by 2013 ESH/ESC guidelines [1]:

RaVL >1.1 mV

Sokolow–Lyon index (S V1-V2 + R V5-V6) >3.8 mV

Cornell voltage duration product (QRS duration * Cornell voltage) >244 mV*ms

B. Other diagnostic criteria

Cornell voltage (S V3 + R aVL) >2.8 mV

Cornell strain (S V3 + R aVL >2.4 mV in male or >2.0 mV in female or ST-segment strain)

Romhilt–Estes ≥4–5 points

Lewis [(R DI + S D III) – (S DI + R DIII)] >1.7 mV

Framingham (ST-segment strain + 1 voltage criterion)

Perugia score (S V3 + R aVL >2.4 mV in male or >2.0 mV in female or ST-segment strain or Romhilt–Estes >5 points)

TABLE 1.2 Echocardiographic criteria for the diagnosis of LV hypertrophy

A. Diagnostic criteria recommended by 2013 ESH/ESC guidelines [1]:

LV mass indexed by body surface area (BSA): men >115 g/m^2; women >95 g/m^2

B. Other diagnostic criteria

LV mass indexed by height$^{2.7}$: >51 $g/m^{2.7}$ (both genders)

Relative wall thickness (RWT): >0.45

echocardiogram, which may provide additional clinical information, including quantitative assessment of LV mass and geometry, LV systolic and diastolic function as well as data on other cardiac chambers (including left atrium and aortic root). All these functional and structural abnormalities may be involved in development and progression of hypertension-induced cardiac remodelling from LV hypertrophy towards LV dysfunction and congestive heart failure.

In this patient, the echocardiographic diagnosis of LV hypertrophy was able to modify his global cardiovascular risk profile from moderate to high, which had important clinical consequences. Indeed, the assessment of cardiac organ damage may help physicians in choosing among different antihypertensive drug classes and tailoring the most effective antihypertensive therapy at appropriate dosages and/or combination, according to compelling indications from current hypertension guidelines [1]. For example, the therapeutic choice for this patient was oriented on a fixed combination therapy based on the angiotensin receptor blocker losartan and the thiazide diuretic hydrochlorothiazide, which has demonstrated beneficial effects on cardiovascular morbidity and mortality in hypertensive patients with LV hypertrophy [7–14].

In the preliminary evaluation of the patient, the main goal of the therapeutic strategy was focused on the correction of modifiable risk factors, including sedentary life habits and visceral overweight. This represents a key element of any antihypertensive therapy at any stage of the disease. In a subsequent step, the discovery of cardiac organ damage induced an up-titration of pharmacological strategy throughout the adoption of antihypertensive drug classes with proven benefits on regression of LV hypertrophy, beyond BP lowering efficacy [7–14].

During the follow-up evaluation of this hypertensive patient with LV hypertrophy, repeated electrocardiographic and/or echocardiographic evaluations of LV mass and geometry may provide indirect evidence of the therapeutic effectiveness of antihypertensive therapy, by demonstrating the regression of LV hypertrophy, a phenomenon that has been associated to a reduced risk of cardiovascular and cerebrovascular complications.

Take-Home Messages

- The presence of cardiac organ damage (namely, LV hypertrophy) increases the risk of developing major cardiovascular and cerebrovascular complications in hypertension.
- The regression of LV hypertrophy, beyond the achievement of effective BP control, has been associated with improved cardiovascular prognosis.
- All hypertensive patients should undergo 12-lead electrocardiogram at first evaluation, in order to assess electrocardiographic criteria for LV hypertrophy.
- In view of the large diffusion, high reproducibility and low cost of electrocardiogram, this exam can be repeated every year, to evaluate potential regression of electrographic criteria of LV hypertrophy.
- Echocardiographic assessment of LV mass and geometry should be limited in those hypertensive patients at medium to high cardiovascular risk, in whom the information obtained by echocardiogram may induce a substantial change in diagnostic and therapeutic approach.
- Advanced diagnostic tests for cardiac organ damage (e.g. magnetic resonance or cardiac CT) should be limited to difficult to treat forms of hypertension and performed in reference centres or excellence centres for hypertension.

References

1. Mancia G, Fagard R, Narkiewicz K, Redon J, Zanchetti A, Bohm M, et al. 2013 ESH/ESC Guidelines for the management of arterial hypertension: the Task Force for the management of arterial hypertension of the European Society of Hypertension (ESH) and of the European Society of Cardiology (ESC). J Hypertens. 2013;31(7):1281–357.
2. Verdecchia P, Dovellini EV, Gorini M, Gozzelino G, Lucci D, Milletich A, et al. Comparison of electrocardiographic criteria for diagnosis of left ventricular hypertrophy in hypertension: the MAVI study. Ital Heart J. 2000;1(3):207–15.
3. Devereux RB, Wallerson DC, de Simone G, Ganau A, Roman MJ. Evaluation of left ventricular hypertrophy by M-mode echocardiography in patients and experimental animals. Am J Card Imaging. 1994;8(4):291–304.
4. Ganau A, Devereux RB, Roman MJ, de Simone G, Pickering TG, Saba PS, et al. Patterns of left ventricular hypertrophy and geometric remodeling in essential hypertension. J Am Coll Cardiol. 1992;19(7):1550–8.
5. de Simone G, Muiesan ML, Ganau A, Longhini C, Verdecchia P, Palmieri V, et al. Reliability and limitations of echocardiographic measurement of left ventricular mass for risk stratification and follow-up in single patients: the RES trial. Working Group on Heart and Hypertension of the Italian Society of Hypertension. Reliability of M-mode Echocardiographic Studies. J Hypertens. 1999;17(12 Pt 2):1955–63.
6. Verdecchia P, Schillaci G, Borgioni C, Ciucci A, Gattobigio R, Zampi I, et al. Prognostic value of a new electrocardiographic method for diagnosis of left ventricular hypertrophy in essential hypertension. J Am Coll Cardiol. 1998;31(2):383–90.
7. Wachtell K, Okin PM, Olsen MH, Dahlof B, Devereux RB, Ibsen H, et al. Regression of electrocardiographic left ventricular hypertrophy during antihypertensive therapy and reduction in sudden cardiac death: the LIFE study. Circulation. 2007;116(7):700–5.
8. Okin PM, Devereux RB, Harris KE, Jern S, Kjeldsen SE, Julius S, et al. Regression of electrocardiographic left ventricular hypertrophy is associated with less hospitalization for heart

failure in hypertensive patients. Ann Intern Med. 2007; 147(5):311–9.

9. Olsen MH, Wachtell K, Ibsen H, Lindholm LH, Dahlof B, Devereux RB, et al. Reductions in albuminuria and in electrocardiographic left ventricular hypertrophy independently improve prognosis in hypertension: the LIFE study. J Hypertens. 2006;24(4):775–81.

10. Okin PM, Wachtell K, Devereux RB, Harris KE, Jern S, Kjeldsen SE, et al. Regression of electrocardiographic left ventricular hypertrophy and decreased incidence of new-onset atrial fibrillation in patients with hypertension. JAMA. 2006;296(10): 1242–8.

11. Okin PM, Devereux RB, Liu JE, Oikarinen L, Jern S, Kjeldsen SE, et al. Regression of electrocardiographic left ventricular hypertrophy predicts regression of echocardiographic left ventricular mass: the LIFE study. J Hum Hypertens. 2004;18(6): 403–9.

12. Okin PM, Devereux RB, Jern S, Kjeldsen SE, Julius S, Nieminen MS, et al. Regression of electrocardiographic left ventricular hypertrophy during antihypertensive treatment and the prediction of major cardiovascular events. JAMA. 2004;292(19): 2343–9.

13. Devereux RB, Dahlof B, Gerdts E, Boman K, Nieminen MS, Papademetriou V, et al. Regression of hypertensive left ventricular hypertrophy by losartan compared with atenolol: the Losartan Intervention for Endpoint Reduction in Hypertension (LIFE) trial. Circulation. 2004;110(11):1456–62.

14. Okin PM, Devereux RB, Jern S, Kjeldsen SE, Julius S, Nieminen MS, et al. Regression of electrocardiographic left ventricular hypertrophy by losartan versus atenolol: the Losartan Intervention for Endpoint reduction in Hypertension (LIFE) study. Circulation. 2003;108(6):684–90.

Clinical Case 2
Patient with Essential Hypertension and Diastolic Dysfunction

2.1 Clinical Case Presentation

A 44-year-old, Caucasian male, officer, presented to the Outpatient Clinic for clinical assessment of uncontrolled essential hypertension.

He has history of essential hypertension by about 15 years. At the first diagnostic examination, all screening tests have excluded secondary forms of hypertension, thus confirming the primary nature of the disease. Then, he was treated with a combination therapy based on ACE inhibitor (enalapril 10 mg) and calcium-channel blocker (nifedipine slow release 30 mg).

About 5 years ago, for incoming lower limb oedema, he was moved to another calcium-channel blocker (from nifedipine SR 30 mg to lercanidipine 10 mg), with satisfactory BP control at home and no relevant side effects or adverse reactions.

By about 8 months, he reported uncontrolled BP levels measured at home and effort dyspnoea. He also described frequent palpitations and tachycardia. For these reasons, his referring physician firstly titrated the dosage of enalapril from 10 to 20 mg daily and then added a thiazide diuretic (hydrochlorothiazide 25 mg daily) to current pharmacological therapy, albeit with limited improvement on BP control and persistent dyspnoea.

G. Tocci, *Hypertension and Organ Damage: A Case-Based Guide to Management*, Practical Case Studies in Hypertension Management, DOI 10.1007/978-3-319-25097-7_2,
© Springer International Publishing Switzerland 2016

Family History

He has paternal history of coronary artery disease and maternal history of hypertension and myocardial infarction. He also has two sisters with hypertension.

Clinical History

He was previously a smoker (more than 20 cigarettes daily) for more than 20 years until the age of 38 years, when chronic obstructive pulmonary disease with a predominant asthmatic component was diagnosed. He also has additional modifiable cardiovascular risk factors, including mild hypercholesterol-emia treated with simvastatin 10 mg daily and hypertriglyc-eridemia treated with fibrates. There are no additional cardiovascular risk factors or concomitant cardiovascular or non-cardiovascular comorbidities.

Physical Examination

- Weight: 87 kg
- Height: 185 cm
- Body mass index (BMI): 25.4 kg/m^2
- Waist circumference: 98 cm
- Respiration: normal
- Heart sounds: distal cardiac sounds with apparently free intervals
- Resting pulse: regular rhythm with normal heart rate (75 beats/min)
- Carotid arteries: no murmurs
- Femoral and foot arteries: palpable

Haematological Profile

- Haemoglobin: 13.8 g/dL
- Haematocrit: 47.2 %

- Fasting plasma glucose: 66 mg/dL
- Fasting lipids: total cholesterol (TOT-C): 169 mg/dl; low-density lipoprotein cholesterol (LDL-C): 105 mg/dl; high-density lipoprotein cholesterol (HDL-C), 43 mg/dl; triglycerides (TG) 104 mg/dl
- Electrolytes: sodium, 141 mEq/L; potassium, 4.3 mEq/L
- Serum uric acid: 3.6 mg/dL
- Renal function: urea, 25 mg/dl; creatinine, 1.2 mg/dL; creatinine clearance (Cockcroft–Gault), 97 ml/min; estimated glomerular filtration rate (eGFR) (MDRD), 75 mL/min/1.73 m^2
- Urine analysis (dipstick): normal
- Albuminuria: 14.7 mg/24 h
- Normal liver function tests
- Normal thyroid function tests

Blood Pressure Profile

- Home BP (average): 150/100 mmHg
- Sitting BP: 153/104 mmHg (right arm); 156/106 mmHg (left arm)
- Standing BP: 157/105 mmHg at 1 min
- 24-h BP: 149/101 mmHg; HR: 67 bpm
- Daytime BP: 135/105 mmHg; HR: 69 bpm
- Night-time BP: 138/92 mmHg; HR: 60 bpm

The 24-h ambulatory blood pressure profile is illustrated in Fig. 2.1.

12-Lead Electrocardiogram

Sinus rhythm with normal heart rate (78 bpm), normal atrio-ventricular conduction with right bundle branch block (Fig. 2.2)

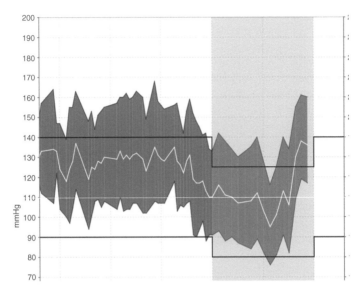

FIGURE 2.1 24-h ambulatory blood pressure profile at first visit

Vascular Ultrasound

Carotid: intima–media thickness at both carotid levels (right: 0.7 mm, and left: 0.8 mm)) without evidence of atherosclerotic plaques

Renal: intima–media thickness at both renal arteries without evidence of atherosclerotic plaques. Normal Doppler examination at both right and left arteries. Normal dimension and structure of the abdominal aorta

Current Treatment

Enalapril 20 mg h 8:00; hydrochlorothiazide 25 mg h 8:00; lercanidipine 10 mg h 20:00

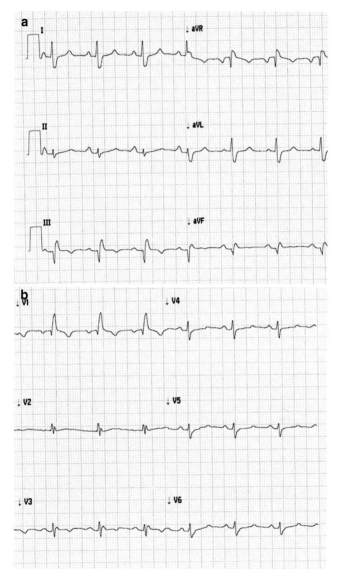

FIGURE 2.2 12-lead electrocardiogram at first visit: sinus rhythm with normal heart rate (78 bpm), normal atrioventricular conduction with right bundle branch block. Peripheral (**a**) and precordial (**b**) leads

Diagnosis

Essential (stage 2) hypertension with unsatisfactory BP control on combination therapy. Additional modifiable cardiovascular risk factors (hypercholesterolemia and hypertriglyceridemia). No evidence of hypertension-related organ damage nor associated clinical conditions.

Which is the global cardiovascular risk profile in this patient?

Possible answers are:

1. Low
2. Medium
3. High
4. Very high

Global Cardiovascular Risk Stratification

According to 2013 ESH/ESC global cardiovascular risk stratification [1], this patient has moderate to high cardiovascular risk.

Which is the best therapeutic option in this patient?

Possible answers are:

1. Add another drug class (e.g. dihydropyridinic calcium antagonist).
2. Add another drug class (e.g. beta-blocker).
3. Switch from ACE inhibitor to ARB combined with thiazide diuretic.
4. Switch from ACE inhibitor to direct renin inhibitor combined with thiazide diuretic.

Treatment Evaluation

- Add beta-blocker at medium dose (atenolol 100 mg ¼ cp h 8:00 and ¼ cp h 20:00).
- Maintain enalapril 20 mg h 8:00, hydrochlorothiazide 25 mg h 8:00 and lercanidipine 10 mg h 20:00.

Prescriptions

- Periodical BP evaluation at home according to recommendations from guidelines
- Echocardiogram aimed at evaluating left ventricular (LV) mass and function (systolic and diastolic properties)

2.2   Follow-Up (Visit 1) at 6 Weeks

At follow-up visit, the patient is in good clinical condition. However, he referred to have prematurely stopped the prescribed therapy with beta-blocker due to perceived deterioration of effort dyspnoea and asthma. He also tried to double the dose of amlodipine 5 mg twice daily, but even in this case, he has to prematurely stop this additional medication due to onset of lower limb oedema and frequent palpitations. For these reasons, he maintained his previous antihypertensive therapy without adverse reactions or drug-related side effects, although the BP levels measured at home remained substantially unchanged.

Physical Examination

- Respiration: normal
- Heart sounds: distal cardiac sounds with apparently free intervals
- Resting pulse: regular rhythm with normal heart rate (74 beats/min)
- Other clinical parameters substantially unchanged

Blood Pressure Profile

- Home BP (average): 150/100 mmHg
- Sitting BP: 154/102 mmHg (right arm); 155/104 mmHg (left arm)
- Standing BP: 156/105 mmHg at 1 min

Current Treatment

Enalapril 20 mg h 8:00; hydrochlorothiazide 25 mg h 8:00; lercanidipine 10 mg h 20:00

Echocardiogram

Concentric remodelling (LV mass indexed 108 g/m^2; relative wall thickness: 0.43) with normal chamber dimension (LV end-diastolic diameter 50 mm) (Fig. 2.3a), impaired LV relaxation at both conventional (E/A ratio <1; Fig. 2.3b) and tissue Doppler evaluations and normal ejection fraction (LV ejection fraction 60 %). In particular, tissue Doppler analysis was performed at both lateral wall of the LV (Fig. 2.3c) and interventricular septum (Fig. 2.3d).

Normal dimension of aortic root and left atrium. Right ventricle with normal dimension and function. Pericardium without relevant abnormalities.

Mitral (+) and tricuspid (+) regurgitations at Doppler ultrasound examination.

Diagnosis

Essential (stage 2) hypertension with unsatisfactory BP control on combination therapy. Initial signs of cardiac organ damage (concentric LV remodelling and impaired LV relaxation). Additional modifiable cardiovascular risk factors (hypercholesterolemia). No associated clinical conditions.

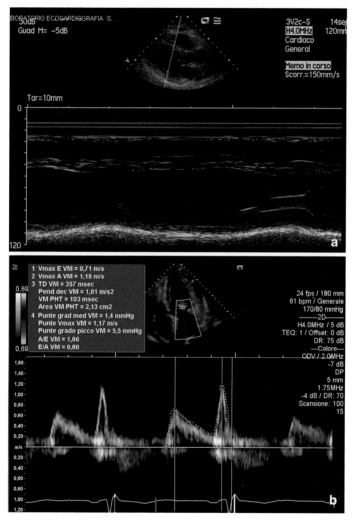

FIGURE 2.3 Echocardiogram at follow-up visit after 6 weeks: concentric remodelling with normal chamber dimension (**a**), impaired LV relaxation at both conventional (**b**) and tissue Doppler evaluations and normal ejection fraction. In particular, tissue Doppler analysis was performed at both lateral wall of the LV (**c**) and interventricular septum (**d**). Normal dimension of aortic root and left atrium. Right ventricle with normal dimension and function. Pericardium without relevant abnormalities

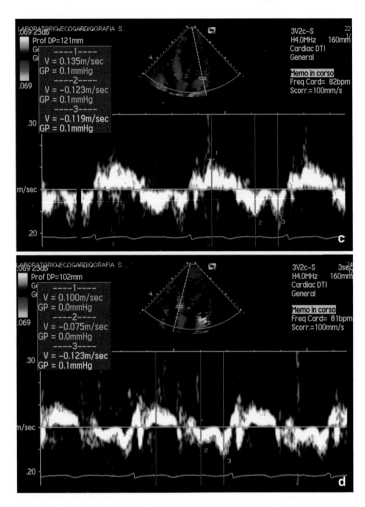

FIGURE 2.3 (continued)

Which is the global cardiovascular risk profile in this patient?

Possible answers are:

1. Low
2. Medium
3. High
4. Very high

Global Cardiovascular Risk Stratification

Echocardiographic evidence of concentric LV remodelling and impaired LV relaxation do not represent a marker of cardiac organ damage, although they can be considered as early structural and functional LV adaptations to abnormal BP load. Thus, this patient remained on moderate to high cardiovascular risk, according to 2013 ESH/ESC global cardiovascular risk stratification [1].

Which is the best therapeutic option in this patient?

Potential answers are:

1. Add another drug class (e.g. dihydropyridinic calcium antagonist).
2. Add another drug class (e.g. beta-blocker).
3. Add another drug class (e.g. alpha-blocker).
4. Switch from ARB to direct renin inhibitor combined with thiazide diuretic.

Treatment Evaluation

- Stop enalapril 20 mg h 8:00.
- Start telmisartan 40 mg h 8:00.
- Maintain hydrochlorothiazide 25 mg h 8:00 and lercanidipine 10 mg h 20:00.

Prescriptions

- Periodical BP evaluation at home according to recommendations from current guidelines

2.3   Follow-Up (Visit 2) at 3 Months

At follow-up visit, the patient is in good clinical condition. He reported good adherence to prescribed medications without adverse reactions or drug-related side effects (absence of dyspnoea and lower limb oedema).

Physical Examination

- Resting pulse: regular rhythm with 67 beats/min
- Other parameters substantially unchanged

Blood Pressure Profile

- Home BP (average): 140/90 mmHg
- Sitting BP: 144/95 mmHg (right arm); 145/93 mmHg (left arm)
- Standing BP: 146/92 mmHg at 1 min

Current Treatment

Telmisartan 40 mg h 8:00; hydrochlorothiazide 25 mg h 8:00; amlodipine 5 mg h 20:00

Which is the best therapeutic option in this patient?
Possible answers are:

1. Add another drug class (e.g. beta-blocker).
2. Add another drug class (e.g. alpha-blocker).
3. Titrate the dosage of current therapy.
4. Switch from ARB to direct renin inhibitor combined with thiazide diuretic.

Treatment Evaluation

- Titrate the dosage of telmisartan from 40 to 80 mg daily and start fixed combination therapy with telmisartan/hydrochlorothiazide 80/25 mg h 8:00.
- Titrate the dosage of lercanidipine from 10 to 20 mg h 20:00.

Prescriptions

- Periodical BP evaluation at home according to recommendations from current guidelines.
- Repeat a 24-h ambulatory BP monitoring to test sustained and effective antihypertensive efficacy of prescribed medications.

2.4 Follow-Up (Visit 2) at 1 Year

At follow-up visit, the patient is in good clinical condition. He also reported good adherence to prescribed medications with no adverse reactions or relevant drug-related side effects.

Physical Examination

- Resting pulse: regular rhythm with 65 beats/min
- Other parameters substantially unchanged

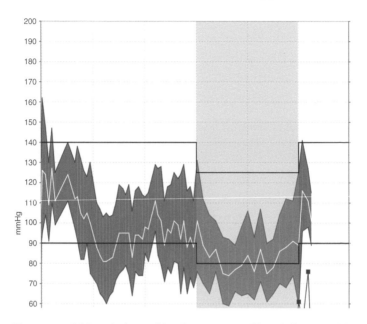

FIGURE 2.4 24-h ambulatory blood pressure profile at follow-up visit after 1 year. Compared to previous examination, 24-h blood pressure profile shows marked reduction of average blood pressure levels, although it can be noted transient blood pressure raises during the first and the last measurements (i.e. white-coat effect)

Blood Pressure Profile

- Home BP (average): 120/80 mmHg
- Sitting BP: 136/82 mmHg (left arm)
- Standing BP: 138/88 mmHg at 1 min
- 24-h BP: 117/77 mmHg; HR: 77 bpm
- Daytime BP: 122/81 mmHg; HR: 82 bpm
- Night-time BP: 104/67 mmHg; HR: 63 bpm

The 24-h ambulatory blood pressure profile is illustrated in Fig. 2.4.

12-Lead Electrocardiogram

Sinus rhythm with normal heart rate (67 bpm), normal atrio-ventricular conduction, right bundle branch block

Current Treatment

Telmisartan/hydrochlorothiazide 80/25 mg h 8:00, lercanidipine 20 mg h 20:00

Treatment Evaluation

- No changes for current pharmacological therapy

Prescriptions

- Periodical BP evaluation at home according to recommendations from current guidelines

**Which is the most useful diagnostic test to repeat
during the follow-up in this patient?**
Possible answers are:

1. Electrocardiogram
2. Echocardiogram
3. Vascular Doppler ultrasound
4. Evaluation of renal parameters (e.g. creatininemia,
   eGFR, ClCr, UACR)
5. 24-h ambulatory BP monitoring

2.5   Discussion

Arterial hypertension is a chronic disease, which promotes the
development and progression of asymptomatic functional and
structural adaptation at cardiac, renal and vascular levels.
Among these, diastolic dysfunction can be viewed as a very
early marker of cardiac organ damage, prior to the development of LV hypertrophy. Even if not always associated with an
increased LV mass, the presence of diastolic dysfunction is able

TABLE 2.1 Echocardiographic criteria for the diagnosis of diastolic dysfunction

	Normal	**Impaired**	**Pseudo-normal**	**Restrictive**
Ratio E/A (trasmitral flow)	>1.0	<1.0	>1.0	≫1.0
Deceleration time (ms)	150–220	>220	150–220	<150
Ratio S/D (pulmonary vein)	>1.0	>1.0	<1.0	≪1.0
Ratio Em/Am	>1.0	<1.0	<1.0	≫1.0
Ratio E/Em	<8	8–12	8–12	≥13
IVRT (ms)	80–100	>100	80–100	<80

IVRT isovolumetric relaxation time

to affect cardiovascular prognosis in hypertensive patients, by increasing the risk of major cardiovascular events [2].

Several diagnostic criteria have been proposed for the echocardiographic assessment of diastolic dysfunction, particularly in the very recent years, in which this condition has been included in the diagnostic work-up of a complex clinical syndrome, that is, "diastolic heart failure" or "heart failure with preserved LV function" (Table 2.1).

In essential hypertension, the presence of diastolic dysfunction is relatively frequent and not always associated with other concomitant cardiac adaptations, mostly including LV hypertrophy [3, 4]. Actually, it has been defined as impaired ratio between early filling phase and atrial contraction during diastole, measured at either conventional Doppler (E/A ratio <1) or tissue Doppler (Em/Am ratio <1) [5].

In this clinical case, some aspects can be discussed. First of all, electrocardiographic evaluation of cardiac organ damage, which represents a fundamental step in the first-line assessment of any patient with hypertension, is of limited efficacy, since the presence of bundle branch block does not allow the proper identification of diagnostic criteria for LV hypertrophy. For this reason, the echocardiographic assessment of LV hypertrophy, as well as LV systolic and diastolic dysfunction, is mandatory, also in view of the presence of effort dyspnoea.

The echocardiographic evaluation of LV geometry reported an increased wall thickness with normal LV chamber dimension and normal LV mass. This condition, defined as LV concentric remodelling, does not represent a "conventional marker" of cardiac organ damage. Although it does not induce any change in the individual global cardiovascular risk profile, it can be viewed as an early larker of the structural and functional LV adaptations, which may lead to further development of LV hypertrophy. In this view, early identification and prompt treatment of this condition may prevent or reduce progression and prevent development of cardiac organ damage.

It should be also noted, however, that diastolic dysfunction as well as LV concentric remodelling do not identify any compelling indication [1]. Hypertension guidelines, in fact, do not consider these cardiac abnormalities as diagnostic elements able to guide physicians in choosing among different antihypertensive drug classes [1].

In this case, the choice of antihypertensive strategy based on a combination therapy with a renin–angiotensin system blocker and a vasodilating agent can be justified by the evidence in favour of these drugs in terms of positive LV remodelling, reduced LV pressure mass and reduced cardiovascular morbidity and mortality, beyond their BP lowering efficacy [6–8].

In the initial evaluation of the patient, the main aspect that conditioned the therapeutic approach was the onset of drug-related side effects, which limited the therapeutic choice to some antihypertensive drug classes or molecules. In a subsequent step, the echocardiographic assessment of diastolic dysfunction associated with LV concentric remodelling and the absence of either global or local impairments of LV systolic properties justified the clinical symptoms (dyspnoea) and were able to orient the therapeutic choices.

As a final consideration, during the follow-up evaluation of this hypertensive patient with diastolic dysfunction, the

24-h ambulatory BP monitoring confirmed the sustained antihypertensive efficacy of the prescribed antihypertensive therapy, beyond clinic and home BP measurements. On the other hand, repeated electrocardiographic assessments are not useful for two main reasons: (1) diastolic dysfunction cannot be assessed by the conventional 12-lead electrocardiogram; (2) the presence of bundle branch block does not allow any comparison with regard to potential changes of LV mass or geometry. Thus, repeated echocardiographic assessment of LV geometry and function represents the only way to able to provide indirect evidence of the therapeutic effectiveness of the prescribed antihypertensive therapy, as also recommended by current guidelines [1].

Take-Home Messages
- Diastolic dysfunction is a relatively frequent condition in hypertensive patients at different cardiovascular risk profile.
- This can be associated with effort dyspnoea and reduced functional capacity, without evidence of (global or local) impairments of LV systolic properties and/or signs or symptoms of congestive heart failure.
- Diastolic dysfunction can be assessed by conventional or tissue Doppler echocardiographic evaluation of the LV properties.
- The presence of diastolic dysfunction, with or without evidence of LV hypertrophy, has been associated with reduced event-free survival and increased risk of major cardiovascular events in essential hypertensive patients.
- Several antihypertensive drug classes (or molecules) have been tested in hypertensive patients with diastolic dysfunction, although limited evidence are available to have definite compelling indications in this clinical setting.

References

1. Mancia G, Fagard R, Narkiewicz K, Redon J, Zanchetti A, Bohm M, et al. 2013 ESH/ESC Guidelines for the management of arterial hypertension: the Task Force for the management of arterial hypertension of the European Society of Hypertension (ESH) and of the European Society of Cardiology (ESC). J Hypertens. 2013;31(7):1281–357.
2. Schillaci G, Pasqualini L, Verdecchia P, Vaudo G, Marchesi S, Porcellati C, et al. Prognostic significance of left ventricular diastolic dysfunction in essential hypertension. J Am Coll Cardiol. 2002;39(12):2005–11.
3. Zanchetti A, Cuspidi C, Comarella L, Rosei EA, Ambrosioni E, Chiariello M, et al. Left ventricular diastolic dysfunction in elderly hypertensives: results of the APROS-diadys study. J Hypertens. 2007;25(10):2158–67.
4. Sciarretta S, Paneni F, Ciavarella GM, De Biase L, Palano F, Baldini R, et al. Evaluation of systolic properties in hypertensive patients with different degrees of diastolic dysfunction and normal ejection fraction. Am J Hypertens. 2009;22(4):437–43.
5. Galderisi M. Diagnosis and management of left ventricular diastolic dysfunction in the hypertensive patient. Am J Hypertens. 2011;24(5):507–17.
6. Takagi H, Mizuno Y, Iwata K, Goto SN, Umemoto T. Blood pressure-independent effects of telmisartan on regression of left ventricular mass: a meta-analysis and meta-regression of randomized controlled trials. Int J Cardiol. 2013;165(3):564–7.
7. Cowan BR, Young AA, Anderson C, Doughty RN, Krittayaphong R, Lonn E, et al. Left ventricular mass and volume with telmisartan, ramipril, or combination in patients with previous atherosclerotic events or with diabetes mellitus (from the ONgoing Telmisartan Alone and in Combination With Ramipril Global Endpoint Trial [ONTARGET]). Am J Cardiol. 2009;104(11): 1484–9.
8. Martina B, Dieterle T, Sigle JP, Surber C, Battegay E. Effects of telmisartan and losartan on left ventricular mass in mild-to-moderate hypertension. A randomized, double-blind trial. Cardiology. 2003;99(3):169–70.

Clinical Case 3
Patient with Essential Hypertension and Microalbuminuria

3.1 Clinical Case Presentation

A 45-year-old, Caucasian female, postal employee, presented to the Outpatient Clinic for recently uncontrolled hypertension.

She has history of essential hypertension and tachycardia by the age of 38 years. She was treated with monotherapy based on beta-blocker (atenololo 100 mg) with initially effective BP control.

By about 3 months, she reported uncontrolled diastolic BP levels measured at work. For this reason, her referring physician prescribed felodipine 10 mg daily in addition to the current pharmacological therapy. However, the patient was not disposed to adding another pill and asked for thorough assessment of her hypertension.

Family History

She has maternal history of hypertension and diabetes.

G. Tocci, *Hypertension and Organ Damage: A Case-Based Guide to Management*, Practical Case Studies in Hypertension Management, DOI 10.1007/978-3-319-25097-7_3,
© Springer International Publishing Switzerland 2016

Clinical History

She is a smoker (about 10 cigarettes daily) for about 15 years, without other additional cardiovascular risk factors, associated clinical conditions or non-cardiovascular diseases.

Physical Examination

- Weight: 58 kg
- Height: 170 cm
- Body mass index (BMI): 20.1 kg/m^2
- Waist circumference: 88 cm
- Respiration: normal
- Heart sounds: S1–S2 regular, normal, systolic murmur at cardiac apex
- Resting pulse: regular rhythm with normal heart rate (65 beats/min)
- Carotid arteries: no murmurs
- Femoral and foot arteries: palpable

Haematological Profile

- Haemoglobin: 16.3 g/dL
- Haematocrit: 52.1 %
- Fasting plasma glucose: 88 mg/dL
- Fasting lipids: total cholesterol (TOT-C), 164 mg/dl; low-density lipoprotein cholesterol (LDL-C), 84 mg/dl; high-density lipoprotein cholesterol (HDL-C), 65 mg/dl; triglycerides (TG) 78 mg/dl
- Electrolytes: sodium, 145 mEq/L; potassium, 4.0 mEq/L
- Serum uric acid: 2.6 mg/dL
- Renal function: urea, 22 mg/dl; creatinine, 1.0 mg/dL; creatinine clearance (Cockcroft–Gault), 77 ml/min; estimated glomerular filtration rate (eGFR) (MDRD), 69 mL/min/1.73 m^2
- Urine analysis (dipstick): proteinuria 20 mg/dl

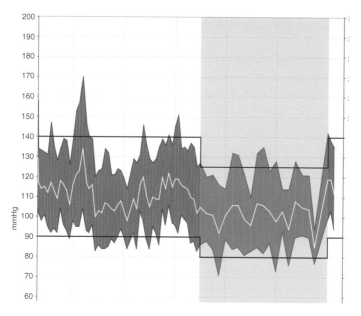

FIGURE 3.1 24-h ambulatory blood pressure profile at first visit

- Normal liver function tests
- Normal thyroid function tests

Blood Pressure Profile

- Home BP (average): 130/100 mmHg
- Sitting BP: 145/98 mmHg (right arm); 142/96 mmHg (left arm)
- Standing BP: 146/95 mmHg at 1 min
- 24-h BP: 131/91 mmHg; HR: 77 bpm
- Daytime BP: 135/93 mmHg; HR: 78 bpm
- Night-time BP: 122/85 mmHg; HR: 75 bpm

The 24-h ambulatory blood pressure profile is illustrated in Fig. 3.1.

12-Lead Electrocardiogram

Sinus rhythm with normal heart rate (65 bpm), normal atrio-ventricular and intraventricular conduction, ST-segment abnormalities without signs of LVH (aVL 0.3 mV; Sokolow–Lyon, 2.7 mV; Cornell voltage, 0.7 mV; Cornel product, 76.3 mV*ms) (Fig. 3.2)

Echocardiogram with Doppler Ultrasound

Normal LV geometry (LV mass indexed 87 g/m²; relative wall thickness: 0.40) with normal chamber dimension (LV end-diastolic diameter 47 mm) (Fig. 3.3a), normal LV relaxation (E/A ratio 1.53) at both conventional (Fig. 3.3b) and tissue (Fig. 3.3c) Doppler evaluation and normal ejection fraction (LV ejection fraction 70 %). Normal dimensions of aortic root and left atrium. Right ventricle with normal dimension and function. Pericardium without relevant abnormalities

Mitral (++) regurgitation at Doppler ultrasound examination

Vascular Ultrasound

Carotid: intima–media thickness at both carotid levels (right: 1.0 mm; left: 1.0 mm) without evidence of atherosclerotic plaques

Renal: intima–media thickness at both renal arteries without evidence of atherosclerotic plaques. Normal Doppler evaluation at both right (Fig. 3.4a) and left (Fig. 3.4b) renal arteries (main vessels and intraparenchymal arteries). Normal dimension and structure of the abdominal aorta

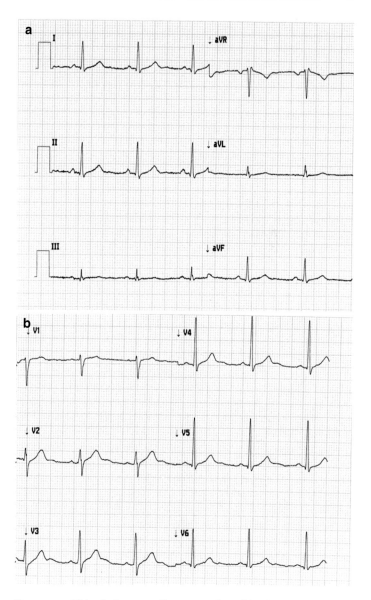

Figure 3.2 12-lead electrocardiogram at first visit: sinus rhythm with normal heart rate (65 bpm), normal atrioventricular and intraventricular conduction, ST-segment abnormalities without signs of LVH. Peripheral (**a**) and precordial (**b**) leads

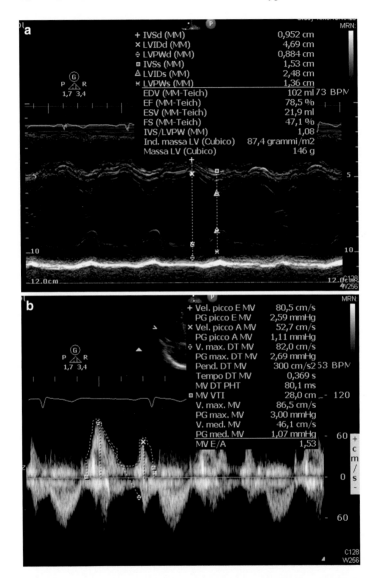

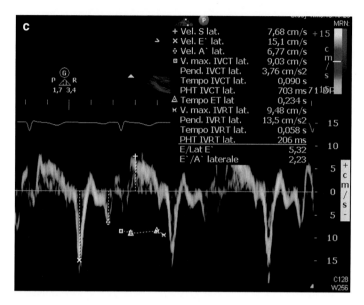

FIGURE 3.3 (continued)

FIGURE 3.3 Echocardiogram with Doppler ultrasound at first visit: normal LV geometry with normal chamber dimension (**a**), normal LV relaxation at both conventional (**b**) and tissue (**c**) Doppler evaluation, and normal ejection fraction. Normal dimensions of aortic root and left atrium. Right ventricle with normal dimension and function. Pericardium without relevant abnormalities

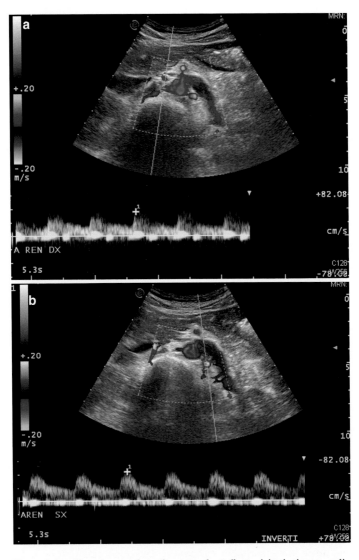

FIGURE 3.4 Renal vascular ultrasound at first visit: intima–media thickness at both renal arteries without evidence of atherosclerotic plaques. Normal Doppler evaluation at both right (**a**) and left (**b**) renal arteries (main vessels and intraparenchymal arteries). Normal dimension and structure of the abdominal aorta

Current Treatment

Atenolol 100 mg ½ cp h 8:00 and ½ cp h 20:00

Diagnosis

Essential (stage 1) hypertension with unsatisfactory BP control on monotherapy. No evidence of hypertension-related organ damage. No additional cardiovascular risk factors nor associated clinical conditions

> **Which is the global cardiovascular risk profile in this patient?**
>
> Possible answers are:
>
> 1. Low
> 2. Medium
> 3. High
> 4. Very high

Global Cardiovascular Risk Stratification

According to 2013 ESH/ESC global cardiovascular risk stratification [1], this patient has low cardiovascular risk.

> **Which is the best therapeutic option in this patient?**
> Possible answers are:
>
> 1. Add another drug class (e.g. dihydropyridinic calcium antagonist).
> 2. Add another drug class (e.g. thiazide diuretic).
> 3. Add another drug class (e.g. ACE inhibitor).
> 4. Add another drug class (e.g. ARB).
> 5. Switch from beta-blocker to another drug class.

Treatment Evaluation

- Gradually stop atenolol 100 mg.
- Start irbesartan 150 mg h 8:00.

Prescriptions

- Periodical BP evaluation at home according to recommendations from guidelines.
- Stop smoking.
- Blood and urinary tests for renal parameters, including serum creatinine, urea estimated glomerular filtration rate and creatinine clearance, and urinary albumin/creatinine ratio on morning urine sample

3.2   Follow-Up (Visit 1) at 6 Weeks

At follow-up visit, the patient is in good clinical condition. She does not stop smoking. However, she reported good adherence to prescribed medications without adverse reactions or drug-related side effects.

Physical Examination

- Resting pulse: regular rhythm with normal heart rate (64 beats/min)
- Other clinical parameters substantially unchanged

Blood Pressure Profile

- Home BP (average): 130/95 mmHg
- Sitting BP: 142/97 mmHg (left arm)
- Standing BP: 144/100 mmHg at 1 min

Current Treatment

Irbesartan 150 mg h 8:00

Haematological Profile

- Electrolytes: sodium, 145 mEq/L; potassium, 3.9 mEq/L
- Renal function: urea, 22 mg/dl, creatinine, 1.05 mg/dL; creatinine clearance (Cockcroft–Gault), 73 ml/min; estimated glomerular filtration rate (eGFR) (MDRD), 65 mL/min/1.73 m^2
- Urine analysis (dipstick): proteinuria 20 mg/dl
- Urinary albumin/creatinine ratio (morning urine sample): 67 mg/g

Diagnosis

Essential (stage 1) hypertension with improved BP control on monotherapy without achieving the recommended BP targets. Renal organ damage (microalbuminuria). No additional cardiovascular risk factors nor associated clinical conditions

Which is the global cardiovascular risk profile in this patient?

Possible answers are:

1. Low
2. Medium
3. High
4. Very high

Global Cardiovascular Risk Stratification

The laboratory evidence of renal organ damage (microalbu-minuria) is able to modify the individual global cardiovascular risk profile. On the basis of this assessment, this patient has moved from low to high cardiovascular risk, according to 2013 ESH/ESC global cardiovascular risk stratification [1]. This would lead to an increased 10-year risk of developing cardiovascular disease (morbidity and mortality).

Which is the best therapeutic option in this patient?

Possible answers are:

1. Add another drug class (e.g. dihydropyridinic calcium antagonist).
2. Add another drug class (e.g. thiazide diuretic).
3. Add another drug class (e.g. ACE inhibitor).
4. Titrate current therapy.

Treatment Evaluation

- Titrate irbesartan from 150 to 300 mg h 8:00.

Prescriptions

- Periodical BP evaluation at home according to recommendations from current guidelines.
- Stop smoking.

3.3   Follow-Up (Visit 2) at 3 Months

At follow-up visit, the patient is in good clinical condition. She reduced smoking consumption to less than 10 cigarettes per week with clinical benefits. She also reported good adherence to prescribed medications without adverse reactions or drug-related side effects.

Physical Examination

- Resting pulse: regular rhythm with 61 beats/min
- Other parameters substantially unchanged

Blood Pressure Profile

- Home BP (average): 130/90 mmHg
- Sitting BP: 138/92 mmHg (left arm)
- Standing BP: 142/93 mmHg at 1 min

Current Treatment

Irbesartan 300 mg h 8:00

Which is the best therapeutic option in this patient?
Possible answers are:

1. Add another drug class (e.g. dihydropyridinic calcium antagonist).
2. Add another drug class (e.g. thiazide diuretic).
3. Add another drug class (e.g. alpha-blocker).
4. Switch from ARB to ACE inhibitor.
5. Switch from ARB to direct renin inhibitor.

Treatment Evaluation

- Add lercanidipine 10 mg h 20:00
- Maintain irbesartan 300 mg h 8:00

Prescriptions

- Periodical BP evaluation at home according to recommendations from current guidelines.
- Stop smoking.
- Blood and urinary tests for renal parameters, including serum creatinine, urea estimated glomerular filtration rate and creatinine clearance, and urinary albumin/creatinine ratio on morning urine sample.
- Repeat the 24-h ambulatory BP monitoring to test sustained and effective antihypertensive efficacy of prescribed medications.

3.4   Follow-Up (Visit 2) at 1 Year

At the follow-up visit, the patient is in good clinical condition. She also reported good adherence to prescribed medications with no adverse reactions or relevant drug-related side effects.

Physical Examination

- Resting pulse: regular rhythm with 65 beats/min
- Other parameters substantially unchanged

Blood Pressure Profile

- Home BP (average): 120/80 mmHg
- Sitting BP: 136/84 mmHg (left arm)
- Standing BP: 137/85 mmHg at 1 min
- 24-h BP: 110/76 mmHg; HR: 63 bpm
- Daytime BP: 114/79 mmHg; HR: 63 bpm
- Night-time BP: 95/65 mmHg; HR: 65 bpm

The 24-h ambulatory blood pressure profile is illustrated in Fig. 3.5.

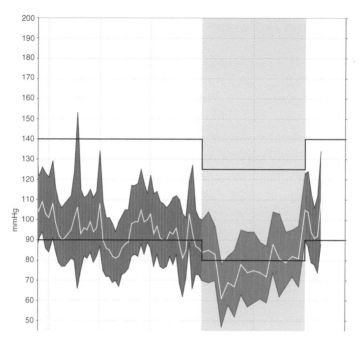

FIGURE 3.5 24-h ambulatory blood pressure profile at follow-up visit after 1 year

Haematological Profile

- Electrolytes: sodium, 146 mEq/L; potassium, 4.1 mEq/L
- Renal function: urea, 23 mg/dl; creatinine, 0.9 mg/dL; creatinine clearance (Cockcroft–Gault), 77 ml/min; estimated glomerular filtration rate (eGFR) (MDRD), 65 mL/min/1.73 m^2
- Urine analysis (dipstick): proteinuria 5 mg/dl
- Urinary albumin/creatinine ratio (morning urine sample): 16 mg/g

Current Treatment

Irbesartan 300 mg h 8:00; lercanidipine 10 mg h 20:00

Treatment Evaluation

- No changes for current pharmacological therapy

Prescriptions

- Periodical BP evaluation at home according to recommendations from current guidelines.
- Stop smoking.

Which is the most useful diagnostic test to repeat during the follow-up in this patient?

Possible answers are:

1. Electrocardiogram
2. Echocardiogram
3. Vascular Doppler ultrasound
4. Evaluation of renal parameters (e.g. creatininemia, eGFR, ClCr, UACR)
5. 24-h ambulatory BP monitoring

3.5   Discussion

The latest sets of hypertension guidelines emphasise the importance of a thorough assessment of hypertension-related organ damage in each individual patient with high BP, as they recognise the beneficial effects in terms of improved cardiovascular prognosis in those hypertensive patients who achieved a delayed progression or even regression of these alterations [2]. In addition, the presence of organ damage is able to help physicians in choosing specific antihypertensive drug classes, which may be more appropriate than others, according to the evidence of compelling indications [2]. Renal organ damage represents today an important marker of disease progression, and it is predictive of future cardiovascular events [3]. For these reasons, accumulating evidence supporting the efficacy of drugs inhibiting the renin–angiotensin system in preventing or delaying the development of renal disease confers to these agents a valuable property that should be considered in the clinical management of hypertension at different cardiovascular risk profile.

In this latter regard, those agents that counteract the effects of the abnormal activation of the renin–angiotensin system, such as ACE inhibitors and angiotensin receptor blockers, have been shown to be effective not only in preventing occurrence or delaying progression but also in promoting regression of hypertension-related organ damage [4]. In particular, both ACE inhibitors and angiotensin receptor blockers are currently recommended to prevent or delay the progression from microalbuminuria to proteinuria and from proteinuria to end-stage renal disease in hypertensive patients with or without diabetes [2].

In this clinical case, some aspects should be discussed. First of all, systematic evaluation of renal organ damage should be always performed at first clinical assessment in all hypertensive patients, in view of its limited cost, large diffusion, simple interpretation and high reproducibility. All these characteristics have been highlighted by the most recent sets of hypertension guidelines, which recommended this examination for guiding both diagnostic and therapeutic decisions in hypertensive patients with or without diabetes [2]. The search for renal organ damage can be integrated by the assessment of serum creatinine levels, estimated glomerular filtration rate, creatinine clearance and dosage of microalbuminuria. Reference values for these parameters are reported on Table 3.1. In particular, microalbuminuria can be assessed either on a 24-h urine collection or morning (spot) sample by testing the urinary albumin/creatinine ratio (UACR). All these functional and structural abnormalities may be involved in development and progression of hypertension-induced renal impairment towards end-stage renal failure.

TABLE 3.1 Diagnostic criteria for the presence of renal organ damage

Serum creatinine: male >115–133 mmol/l (1.3–1.5 mg/dl); female: 107–124 mmol/l (1.2–1.4 mg/dl)

Low estimated glomerular filtration rate by MDRD formula (<60 ml/min/1.73 m^2)

Low estimated glomerular filtration rate by creatinine clearance by Cockcroft–Gault formula (<60 ml/min).

Dosage of microalbuminuria at a 24-h urine sample: 30–300 mg/24 h

Urine albumin–creatinine ratio [UACR] at morning urine sample: male >22; female >31 mg/g creatinine

In this patient, the presence of microalbuminuria was able to modify her global cardiovascular risk profile from moderate to high, which had important clinical consequences. Indeed, the presence of renal organ damage may help physicians in choosing among different antihypertensive drug classes and adopting the most effective antihypertensive therapy at appropriate dosages and/or combination, according to compelling indications from current hypertension guidelines [1]. For example, the therapeutic choice for this patient was a combination therapy based on the angiotensin receptor blocker irbesartan, which has demonstrated beneficial effects on cardiovascular morbidity and mortality in hypertensive patients with microalbuminuria [5–7].

In the preliminary evaluation of the patient, the main goal of the therapeutic strategy was focused on the proper assessment of individual global cardiovascular risk profile. In a subsequent step, the discovery of renal organ damage induced an up-titration of pharmacological strategy throughout the adoption of antihypertensive drug classes with proven benefits on regression of microalbuminuria, beyond BP lowering efficacy [5–7].

During the follow-up evaluation of this hypertensive patient with microalbuminuria, repeated evaluations of renal parameters may provide indirect evidence of the therapeutic effectiveness of antihypertensive therapy, by demonstrating the regression of renal impairment, a phenomenon that has been associated to a reduced risk of cardiovascular, cerebrovascular and renal complications [5–7].

> **Take-Home Messages**
> - Microalbuminuria is a relatively common condition in hypertensive patients at different cardiovascular risk profile, with or without diabetes.
> - This can be associated with impaired renal function, with or without evidence of abnormal serum creatinine levels, estimated glomerular filtration rate and/or creatinine clearance.
> - Microalbuminuria can be assessed by a 24-h urine collection or morning (spot) sample; the preferred diagnostic test should be the urinary albumin/creatinine ratio (UACR).
> - The presence of microalbuminuria has been strongly and independently associated with increased risk of major cardiovascular events, as well as renal failure in essential hypertensive patients.
> - Several antihypertensive drug classes (or molecules) have been tested in hypertensive patients with microalbuminuria, although those drugs able to counteract the renin–angiotensin system, including ACE inhibitors and angiotensin receptor blockers, should be preferred in this clinical setting.

References

1. Mancia G, Fagard R, Narkiewicz K, Redon J, Zanchetti A, Bohm M, et al. 2013 ESH/ESC Guidelines for the management of arterial hypertension: the Task Force for the management of arterial hypertension of the European Society of Hypertension (ESH) and of the European Society of Cardiology (ESC). J Hypertens. 2013;31(7):1281–357.
2. Mancia G, De Backer G, Dominiczak A, Cifkova R, Fagard R, Germano G, et al. 2007 ESH-ESC practice guidelines for the

management of arterial hypertension: ESH-ESC task force on the management of arterial hypertension. J Hypertens. 2007; 25(9):1751–62.

3. Redon J. Treatment of patients with essential hypertension and microalbuminuria. Drugs. 1997;54(6):857–66.

4. Volpe M. Microalbuminuria screening in patients with hypertension: recommendations for clinical practice. Int J Clin Pract. 2008;62(1):97–108.

5. Massie BM, Carson PE, McMurray JJ, Komajda M, McKelvie R, Zile MR, et al. Irbesartan in patients with heart failure and preserved ejection fraction. N Engl J Med. 2008;359(23):2456–67.

6. Parving HH, Lehnert H, Brochner-Mortensen J, Gomis R, Andersen S, Arner P. The effect of irbesartan on the development of diabetic nephropathy in patients with type 2 diabetes. N Engl J Med. 2001;345(12):870–8.

7. Lewis EJ, Hunsicker LG, Clarke WR, Berl T, Pohl MA, Lewis JB, et al. Renoprotective effect of the angiotensin-receptor antagonist irbesartan in patients with nephropathy due to type 2 diabetes. N Engl J Med. 2001;345(12):851–60.

Clinical Case 4
Patient with Essential Hypertension and Proteinuria

4.1 Clinical Case Presentation

A 67-year-old, Caucasian female, teaching professor at the University of Ancient Literature, presented to the Outpatient Clinic for uncontrolled hypertension.

She has history of essential hypertension by about 20 years, treated with ACE inhibitor (ramipril 10 mg), beta-blockers and thiazide diuretic (nebivolol 5/25 mg) with satisfactory BP control.

By about 3 months, she reported uncontrolled BP levels measured at work. For this reason, her referring physician prescribed a calcium-channel blocker (lacidipine 6 mg) in addition to current pharmacological therapy.

Family History

He has maternal history of hypertension and diabetes and paternal history of coronary artery disease and diabetes.

Clinical History

She is a smoker (about 20 cigarettes daily) by more than 20 years. She is affected by dyslipidaemia, treated with combination therapy of simvastatin/ezetimibe 20/10 mg daily. She also

G. Tocci, *Hypertension and Organ Damage: A Case-Based Guide to Management*, Practical Case Studies in Hypertension Management, DOI 10.1007/978-3-319-25097-7_4,
© Springer International Publishing Switzerland 2016

reported intense working activity and mental stress with limited physical activity. About 5 years ago, she started metformin 1000 mg for impaired fasting glucose. She has no other additional cardiovascular risk factors, associated clinical conditions or non-cardiovascular diseases.

Physical Examination

- Weight: 77 kg
- Height: 175 cm
- Body mass index (BMI): 24.1 kg/m^2
- Waist circumference: 97 cm
- Respiration: normal
- Heart sounds: S1–S2 regular, normal, no murmurs
- Resting pulse: regular rhythm with normal heart rate (60 beats/min)
- Carotid arteries: no murmurs
- Femoral and foot arteries: palpable

Haematological Profile

- Haemoglobin: 15.7 g/dL
- Haematocrit: 54.5 %
- Fasting plasma glucose: 73 mg/dL
- Fasting lipids: total cholesterol (TOT-C), 196 mg/dl; low-density lipoprotein cholesterol (LDL-C), 140 mg/dl; high-density lipoprotein cholesterol (HDL-C), 28 mg/dl; triglycerides (TG) 140 mg/dl
- Electrolytes: sodium, 141 mEq/L; potassium, 4.4 mEq/L
- Serum uric acid: 5.8 mg/dL
- Renal function: urea, 28 mg/dl; creatinine 1.08 mg/dL; creatinine clearance (Cockcroft–Gault), 61 ml/mn; estimated glomerular filtration rate (eGFR) (MDRD), 54 mL/min/1.73 m^2
- Urine analysis (dipstick): proteinuria 20 mg/dl
- Normal liver function tests
- Normal thyroid function tests

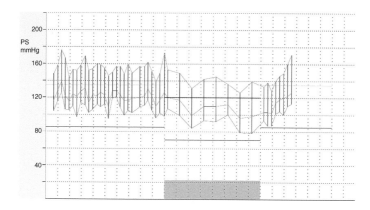

FIGURE 4.1 24-h ambulatory blood pressure profile at first visit

Blood Pressure Profile

- Home BP (average): 140/100 mmHg
- Sitting BP: 155/108 mmHg (right arm); 152/106 mmHg (left arm)
- Standing BP: 156/105 mmHg at 1 min
- 24-h BP: 151/103 mmHg; HR: 75 bpm
- Daytime BP: 153/106 mmHg; HR: 78 bpm
- Night-time BP: 140/92 mmHg; HR: 62 bpm

The 24-h ambulatory blood pressure profile is illustrated in Fig. 4.1.

12-Lead Electrocardiogram

Sinus rhythm with normal heart rate (69 bpm), normal atrio-ventricular and intraventricular conduction, ST-segment abnormalities without signs of LVH (aVL 0.7 mV; Sokolow–Lyon, 2.2 mV; Cornell voltage 1.2 mV; Cornell product 99.6 mV*ms) (Fig. 4.2)

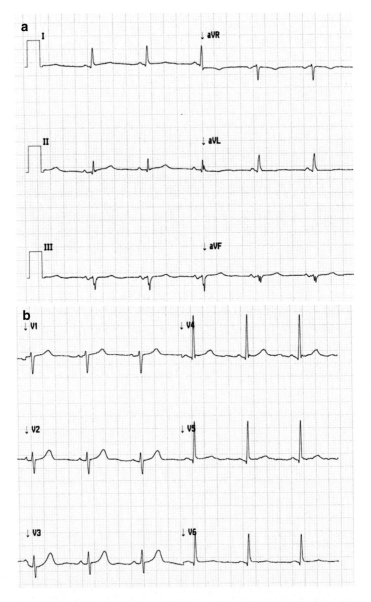

FIGURE 4.2 12-lead electrocardiogram at first visit: sinus rhythm with normal heart rate (69 bpm), normal atrioventricular and intraventricular conduction, ST-segment abnormalities without signs of LVH. Peripheral (**a**) and precordial (**b**) leads

Echocardiogram with Doppler Ultrasound

Concentric LV remodelling (LV mass indexed 93 g/m²; relative wall thickness: 0.47) with normal chamber dimension (LV end-diastolic diameter 44 mm) (Fig. 4.3a), impaired LV relaxation (E/A ratio 1.02) (Fig. 4.3b) at conventional Doppler evaluation and normal ejection fraction (LV ejection fraction 60 %). Normal dimensions of aortic root and left atrium. Right ventricle with normal dimension and function. Pericardium without relevant abnormalities

Mitral (+) regurgitation at Doppler ultrasound examination

Vascular Ultrasound

Carotid: intima–media thickness at both carotid levels (right: 1.1 mm; left: 1.2 mm) without evidence of atherosclerotic plaques

Renal: intima–media thickness at both renal arteries without evidence of atherosclerotic plaques. Normal Doppler evaluation at both right (Fig. 4.4a) and left (Fig. 4.4b) renal arteries. Normal dimension and structure of the abdominal aorta

Current Treatment

Ramipril 10 mg h 8:00; nebivolol 5/25 mg h 8:00; lacidipine 6 mg h 20:00; metformin 500 mg h 12:00 and h 20:00; aspirin 100 mg h 12:00; simvastatin/ezetimibe 20/10 mg h 22:00

Diagnosis

Essential (stage 2) hypertension with unsatisfactory BP control on combination therapy. Smoking, dyslipidaemia, impaired glucose tolerance, sedentary life with work-related stress. Renal impairment (eGFR <60 mL/min/1.73 m² with

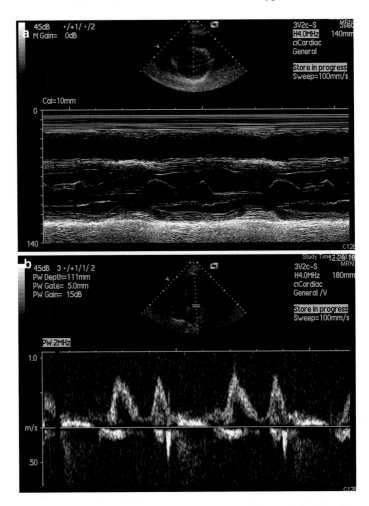

FIGURE 4.3 Echocardiogram with Doppler ultrasound at first visit: concentric LV remodelling with normal chamber dimension (**a**), impaired LV relaxation (**b**) at conventional Doppler evaluation and normal ejection fraction. Normal dimensions of aortic root and left atrium. Right ventricle with normal dimension and function. Pericardium without relevant abnormalities. Mitral (+) regurgitation at Doppler ultrasound examination

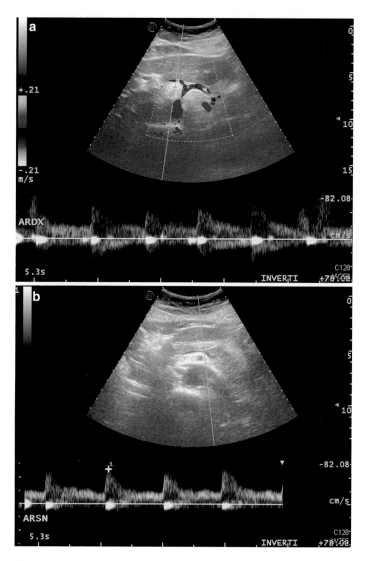

FIGURE 4.4 Renal vascular ultrasound at first visit: intima–media thickness at both renal arteries without evidence of atherosclerotic plaques. Normal Doppler evaluation at both right (**a**) and left (**b**) renal arteries. Normal dimension and structure of the abdominal aorta

normal creatinine clearance). No evidence of cardiac and vascular organ damage. No other additional cardiovascular risk factors nor associated clinical conditions

Which is the global cardiovascular risk profile in this patient?

Possible answers are:

1. Low
2. Medium
3. High
4. Very high

Global Cardiovascular Risk Stratification

According to 2013 ESH/ESC global cardiovascular risk stratification [1], this patient has high cardiovascular risk.

Which is the best therapeutic option in this patient?

Possible answers are:

1. Add another drug class (e.g. antialdosterone agent).
2. Add another drug class (e.g. loop diuretic).
3. Add another drug class (e.g. alpha-blocker).
4. Switch from ACE inhibitor to angiotensin receptor blocker.
5. Switch from ACE inhibitor to direct renin inhibitor.

Treatment Evaluation

- Stop ramipril 10 mg and start valsartan 80 mg h 8:00.
- Stop lacidipine 6 mg and start amlodipine 5 mg h 20:00.
- Maintain nebivolol 5/25 mg h 8:00, metformin 500 mg h 12:00 and h 20:00, aspirin 100 mg h 12:00 and simvastatin/ezetimibe 20/10 mg h 22:00.

Prescriptions

- Periodical BP evaluation at home according to recommendations from guidelines.
- Stop smoking.
- Try to reduce work overload and physical stress.
- Moderate physical activity.
- Blood and urinary tests for renal parameters, including serum creatinine, urea estimated glomerular filtration rate and creatinine clearance, and urinary albumin/creatinine ratio on morning urine sample.

4.2   Follow-Up (Visit 1) at 6 Weeks

At follow-up visit, the patient is in good clinical condition. She does not stop smoking. However, she reported reduced work stress and good adherence to prescribed medications without adverse reactions or drug-related side effects.

Physical Examination

- Resting pulse: regular rhythm with normal heart rate (64 beats/min)
- Other clinical parameters substantially unchanged

Blood Pressure Profile

- Home BP (average): 140/95 mmHg
- Sitting BP: 148/101 mmHg (left arm)
- Standing BP: 146/102 mmHg at 1 min

Current Treatment

Valsartan 80 mg h 8:00; nebivolol 5/25 mg h 8:00; amlodipine 5 mg h 20:00; metformin 500 mg h 12:00 and h 20:00; aspirin 100 mg h 12:00; simvastatin/ezetimibe 20/10 mg h 22:00

Haematological Profile

- Electrolytes: sodium, 143 mEq/L; potassium, 4.2 mEq/L
- Renal function: urea, 27 mg/dl, creatinine, 1.06 mg/dL; creatinine clearance (Cockcroft–Gault), 74 ml/mn; estimated glomerular filtration rate (eGFR) (MDRD), 59 mL/min/1.73 m^2
- Urine analysis (dipstick): proteinuria 20 mg/dl
- Urinary albumin/creatinine ratio (morning urine sample): 82 mg/g

Diagnosis

Essential (stage 2) hypertension with improved BP control on combination therapy without achieving the recommended BP targets. Smoking, dyslipidaemia, impaired glucose tolerance, sedentary life with work-related stress. Renal organ damage (proteinuria). No evidence of cardiac and vascular organ damage. No other additional cardiovascular risk factors nor associated clinical conditions

Which is the global cardiovascular risk profile in this patient?

Possible answers are:

1. Low
2. Medium
3. High
4. Very high

Global Cardiovascular Risk Stratification

The laboratory evidence of proteinuria confirms the presence of renal organ damage. According to 2013 ESH/ESC global cardiovascular risk stratification [1], this patient has high cardiovascular risk. This would lead to an increased 10-year risk of developing cardiovascular disease (morbidity and mortality).

Which is the best therapeutic option in this patient?
Possible answers are:

1. Add another drug class (e.g. antialdosterone agent).
2. Add another drug class (e.g. loop diuretic).
3. Add another drug class (e.g. alpha-blocker).
4. Switch from angiotensin receptor blocker to direct renin inhibitor.
5. Titrate current therapy.

Treatment Evaluation

- Titrate valsartan from 80 mg to 160 mg h 8:00.
- Maintain nebivolol 5/25 mg h 8:00, amlodipine 5 mg h 20:00, metformin 500 mg h 12:00 and h 20:00, aspirin 100 mg h 12:00 and simvastatin/ezetimibe 20/10 mg h 22:00.

Prescriptions

- Periodical BP evaluation at home according to recommendations from guidelines.
- Stop smoking.
- Try to reduce work overload and physical stress.
- Moderate physical activity.
- Blood and urinary tests for renal parameters, including serum creatinine, urea estimated glomerular filtration rate and creatinine clearance, and urinary albumin/creatinine ratio on morning urine sample.

4.3   Follow-Up (Visit 2) at 3 Months

At follow-up visit, the patient is in good clinical condition. She reduced smoking consumption to less than 15 cigarettes per week. She also reported good adherence to prescribed medications without adverse reactions or drug-related side effects.

Physical Examination

- Resting pulse: regular rhythm with 62 beats/min
- Other parameters substantially unchanged

Blood Pressure Profile

- Home BP (average): 135/90 mmHg
- Sitting BP: 143/96 mmHg (left arm)
- Standing BP: 144/94 mmHg at 1 min

Current Treatment

Valsartan 160 mg h 8:00; nebivolol 5/25 mg h 8:00; amlodipine 5 mg h 20:00; metformin 500 mg h 12:00 and h 20:00; aspirin 100 mg h 12:00; simvastatin/ezetimibe 20/10 mg h 22:00

Haematological Profile

- Renal function: urea, 26 mg/dl; creatinine, 1.05 mg/dL; creatinine clearance (Cockcroft–Gault), 74 ml/mn; estimated glomerular filtration rate (eGFR) (MDRD), 60 mL/min/1.73 m^2
- Urinary albumin/creatinine ratio (morning urine sample): 64 mg/g

Which is the best therapeutic option in this patient?

Possible answers are:

1. Add another drug class (e.g. antialdosterone agent).
2. Add another drug class (e.g. loop diuretic).
3. Add another drug class (e.g. alpha-blocker).
4. Switch from angiotensin receptor blocker to direct renin inhibitor.
5. Titrate current therapy.

Treatment Evaluation

- Titrate valsartan from 160 mg to 320 mg h 8:00.
- Maintain nebivolol 5/25 mg h 8:00, lacidipine 6 mg h 20:00, metformin 500 mg h 12:00 and h 20:00, aspirin 100 mg h 12:00 and simvastatin/ezetimibe 20/10 mg h 22:00.

Prescriptions

- Periodical BP evaluation at home according to recommendations from current guidelines.
- Stop smoking.
- Blood and urinary tests for renal parameters, including serum creatinine, urea estimated glomerular filtration rate and creatinine clearance, and urinary albumin/creatinine ratio on morning urine sample.
- Repeat the 24-h ambulatory BP monitoring to test sustained and effective antihypertensive efficacy of prescribed medications.

4.4   Follow-Up (Visit 2) at 1 Year

At follow-up visit, the patient is in good clinical condition. She has further reduced smoking consumption to less than 10 cigarettes daily. She also reported good adherence to prescribed medications with no adverse reactions or relevant drug-related side effects.

Physical Examination

- Resting pulse: regular rhythm with 64 beats/min
- Other parameters substantially unchanged

Blood Pressure Profile

- Home BP (average): 130/80 mmHg
- Sitting BP: 138/86 mmHg (left arm)

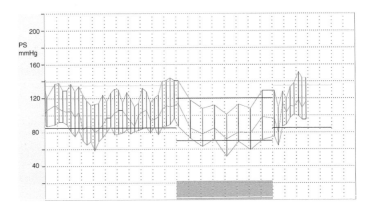

FIGURE 4.5   24-h ambulatory blood pressure profile at follow-up visit after 1 year

- Standing BP: 137/87 mmHg at 1 min
- 24-h BP: 126/81 mmHg; HR: 83 bpm
- Daytime BP: 128/83 mmHg; HR: 85 bpm
- Night-time BP: 116/68 mmHg; HR: 75 bpm

The 24-h ambulatory blood pressure profile is illustrated in Fig. 4.5.

Haematological Profile

- Renal function: urea, 24 mg/dl; creatinine, 1.0 mg/dL; creatinine clearance (Cockcroft–Gault), 78 ml/min; estimated glomerular filtration rate (eGFR) (MDRD), 64 mL/min/1.73 m^2
- Urine analysis (dipstick): proteinuria 5 mg/dl
- Urinary albumin/creatinine ratio (morning urine sample): 18 mg/g

Current Treatment

Valsartan 320 mg h 8:00; nebivolol 5/25 mg h 8:00; amlodipine 5 mg h 20:00; metformin 500 mg h 12:00 and h 20:00; aspirin 100 mg h 12:00; simvastatin/ezetimibe 20/10 mg h 22:00

Treatment Evaluation

- Start fixed combination therapy with valsartan/amlodipine 320/5 mg h 20:00.
- Maintain nebivolol 5/25 mg h 8:00, metformin 500 mg h 12:00 and h 20:00, aspirin 100 mg h 12:00 and simvastatin/ezetimibe 20/10 mg h 22:00.

Prescriptions

- Periodical BP evaluation at home according to recommendations from current guidelines.
- Stop smoking.

Which is the most useful diagnostic test to repeat during the follow-up in this patient?

Possible answers are:

1. Electrocardiogram
2. Echocardiogram
3. Vascular Doppler ultrasound
4. Evaluation of renal parameters (e.g. creatininemia, eGFR, ClCr, UACR)
5. 24-h ambulatory BP monitoring

4.5   Discussion

The clinical relevance of renal organ damage, also in hypertensive patients with or without diabetes, has been recently reaffirmed by the most recent sets of hypertension guidelines, which emphasise the importance of a thorough assessment of hypertension-related organ damage in each individual patient with hypertension [2]. Among various markers of hypertension-related organ damage, renal abnormalities can be now viewed as an important marker of the disease, mostly in view of its predictive value of future cardiovascular and renal events, as well as its high sensitivity for drug-induced changes over time [2]. These aspects have been highlighted by current guidelines, which promoted the systematic search of renal abnormalities in all hypertensive patients, both at first diagnostic evaluation and during the follow-up.

A large body of evidence convincingly and independently demonstrated the antihypertensive efficacy and the favourable effects in terms of reduced cardiovascular and renal complications of drugs inhibiting the renin–angiotensin system in hypertensive patients with renal disease [3–7]. These evidence have demonstrated that both ACE inhibitors and angiotensin receptor are able to prevent or delay the development of renal damage in hypertensive patients at different risk profile [3–7]. For these reasons, both ACE inhibitors and angiotensin receptor blockers are currently recommended to prevent or delay the progression from microalbuminuria to proteinuria and from proteinuria to end-stage renal disease in hypertensive patients with or without diabetes [2].

In this clinical case, some aspects should be discussed. First of all, systematic evaluation of renal organ damage should be always performed at first clinical assessment in all hypertensive patients, in view of its limited cost, large diffusion, simple interpretation and high reproducibility. All these characteristics have been highlighted by the most recent sets of hypertension guidelines, which recommended this examination for guiding both diagnostic and therapeutic decisions in hypertensive patients with or without diabetes [2]. The search for renal organ damage can be integrated by the assessment of serum creatinine levels, estimated glomerular filtration rate, creatinine clearance and dosage of microalbuminuria. All these functional and structural abnormalities may be involved in the development and progression of hypertension-induced renal impairment towards end-stage renal failure.

In this patient with uncontrolled BP levels on combination therapy, the concomitant presence of multiple cardiovascular risk factors and signs of early renal impairment (reduced eGFR with normal creatinine clearance) conferred a high global cardiovascular risk profile. So why perform an additional test to exclude the presence of proteinuria? The most appropriate reason which may explain this decision was related not only to confirming the presence of renal organ damage but mostly to the quantitative assessment of this marker of hypertension-related organ damage, which had important clinical consequences. Indeed, the baseline assessment of proteinuria can provide relevant clinical information during the follow-up presence of these high-risk hypertensive patients. In fact, monitoring the changes of proteinuria over time may provide and indirectly measure the antihypertensive efficacy of the prescribed medications.

In fact, the presence of renal organ damage may help physicians in choosing among different antihypertensive drug classes and adopting the most effective antihypertensive therapy at appropriate dosages and/or combination, according to compelling indications from current hypertension guidelines [1]. For example, the therapeutic choice for this patient was a combination therapy based on the angiotensin receptor blocker valsartan and the calcium-channel blocker amlodipine, which have demonstrated beneficial effects on cardiovascular morbidity and mortality in hypertensive patients with renal disease, with or without diabetes [3–7].

In the preliminary evaluation of the patient, the main goal of the therapeutic strategy was focused on the proper assessment of individual global cardiovascular risk profile. In a subsequent step, the discovery of renal organ damage induced an up-titration of pharmacological strategy throughout the adoption of antihypertensive drug classes with proven benefits on regression of microalbuminuria, beyond BP lowering efficacy [3–7].

During the follow-up evaluation of this hypertensive patient with proteinuria, repeated evaluations of renal parameters provided indirect evidence of the therapeutic effectiveness of antihypertensive therapy, by demonstrating the regression of renal impairment, a phenomenon that has been associated to a reduced risk of cardiovascular and cerebrovascular [3–7].

Take-Home Messages

- Proteinuria is a marker of renal organ damage in hypertensive patients, with or without diabetes, at different cardiovascular risk profile.
- This can be associated with impaired renal function, with or without evidence of abnormal serum creatinine levels, estimated glomerular filtration rate and/or creatinine clearance.
- Proteinuria can be assessed by a 24-h urine collection or morning (spot) sample; the preferred diagnostic test should be the urinary albumin/creatinine ratio (UACR).
- The presence of proteinuria has been strongly and independently associated with increased risk of major cardiovascular and cerebrovascular events, as well as progression towards end-stage renal disease in hypertensive patients at different cardiovascular risk profile.
- Several antihypertensive drug classes (or molecules) have been tested in hypertensive patients with proteinuria, although those drugs able to counteract the renin–angiotensin system, including ACE inhibitors and angiotensin receptor blockers, should be preferred in this clinical setting.

References

1. Mancia G, Fagard R, Narkiewicz K, Redon J, Zanchetti A, Bohm M, et al. 2013 ESH/ESC Guidelines for the management of arterial hypertension: the Task Force for the management of arterial hypertension of the European Society of Hypertension (ESH) and of the European Society of Cardiology (ESC). J Hypertens. 2013;31(7):1281–357.
2. Mancia G, De Backer G, Dominiczak A, Cifkova R, Fagard R, Germano G, et al. 2007 ESH-ESC practice guidelines for the management of arterial hypertension: ESH-ESC task force on

the management of arterial hypertension. J Hypertens. 2007; 25(9):1751–62.

3. Parving HH, Lehnert H, Brochner-Mortensen J, Gomis R, Andersen S, Arner P. The effect of irbesartan on the development of diabetic nephropathy in patients with type 2 diabetes. N Engl J Med. 2001;345(12):870–8.

4. Brenner BM, Cooper ME, de Zeeuw D, Keane WF, Mitch WE, Parving HH, et al. Effects of losartan on renal and cardiovascular outcomes in patients with type 2 diabetes and nephropathy. N Engl J Med. 2001;345(12):861–9.

5. Lewis EJ, Hunsicker LG, Clarke WR, Berl T, Pohl MA, Lewis JB, et al. Renoprotective effect of the angiotensin-receptor antagonist irbesartan in patients with nephropathy due to type 2 diabetes. N Engl J Med. 2001;345(12):851–60.

6. Lindholm LH, Ibsen H, Dahlof B, Devereux RB, Beevers G, de Faire U, et al. Cardiovascular morbidity and mortality in patients with diabetes in the Losartan Intervention For Endpoint reduction in hypertension study (LIFE): a randomised trial against atenolol. Lancet. 2002;359(9311):1004–10.

7. Haller H, Ito S, Izzo Jr JL, Januszewicz A, Katayama S, Menne J, et al. Olmesartan for the delay or prevention of microalbuminuria in type 2 diabetes. N Engl J Med. 2011;364(10):907–17.

Clinical Case 5
Patient with Essential Hypertension and Atherosclerosis

5.1 Clinical Case Presentation

A 77-year-old, Caucasian female, housewife, presented to the Outpatient Clinic for recently uncontrolled hypertension.

She has history of essential hypertension by more than 30 years, treated with combination therapy with beta-blocker and thiazide diuretic (nebivolol/HCTZ 5/12.5 mg) and ACE inhibitor (lisinopril 10 mg).

By about 6 months, she reported uncontrolled BP levels measured at home and at general practitioner. For this reason, her referring physician firstly titrated the dosage of thiazide diuretic from 12.5 to 25 mg combined with the beta-blocker nebivolol 5 mg and the prescribed a dihydropyridinic calcium-channel blocker (lacidipine 6 mg daily) in addition to current pharmacological therapy. However, the patient referred persistently high BP levels at home; she also described a relatively frequent missing assumption of some drugs, due to high pills' burden.

Family History

She has paternal history of hypertension and stroke and maternal history of dyslipidaemia.

G. Tocci, *Hypertension and Organ Damage: A Case-Based Guide to Management*, Practical Case Studies in Hypertension Management, DOI 10.1007/978-3-319-25097-7_5,
© Springer International Publishing Switzerland 2016

Clinical History

She was previous a smoker by more than 35 years (20 cigarettes daily). She was affected by hypercholesterolaemia initially treated with atorvastatin 20–40 mg and now treated
with rosuvastatin 5 mg daily. There are no other additional
cardiovascular risk factors, associated clinical conditions or
non-cardiovascular diseases.

Physical Examination

- Weight: 55 kg
- Height: 160 cm
- Body mass index (BMI): 21.5 kg/m^2
- Waist circumference: 88 cm
- Respiration: normal
- Heart sounds: S1–S2 regular, normal, no murmurs
- Resting pulse: regular rhythm with normal heart rate
  (68 beats/min)
- Carotid arteries: right bruit
- Femoral and foot arteries: palpable

Haematological Profile

- Haemoglobin: 15.0 g/dL
- Haematocrit: 54.7 %
- Fasting plasma glucose: 91 mg/dL
- Fasting lipids: total cholesterol (TOT-C), 186 mg/dl; low-
  density lipoprotein cholesterol (LDL-C), 126 mg/dl; high-
  density lipoprotein cholesterol (HDL-C), 44 mg/dl;
  triglycerides (TG) 132 mg/dl
- Electrolytes: sodium, 146 mEq/L; potassium, 4.1 mEq/L
- Serum uric acid: 4.1 mg/dL
- Renal function: urea, 20 mg/dl; creatinine, 0.5 mg/dL; creati-
  nine clearance (Cockcroft–Gault), 81 ml/mn; estimated glo-
  merular filtration rate (eGFR) (MDRD), 129 mL/min/1.73 m^2
- Urine analysis (dipstick): proteinuria 5 mg/dl

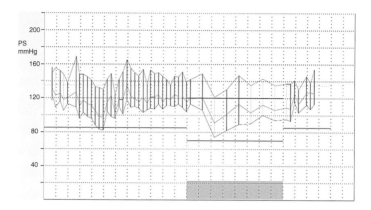

Figure 5.1 24-h ambulatory blood pressure profile at first visit

- Normal liver function tests
- Normal thyroid function tests

Blood Pressure Profile

- Home BP (average): 150/100 mmHg
- Sitting BP: 145/106 mmHg (right arm); 144/108 mmHg (left arm)
- Standing BP: 151/107 mmHg at 1 min
- 24-h BP: 144/104 mmHg; HR: 77 bpm
- Daytime BP: 145/106 mmHg; HR: 79 bpm
- Night-time BP: 138/94 mmHg; HR: 65 bpm

The 24-h ambulatory blood pressure profile is illustrated in Fig. 5.1.

12-Lead Electrocardiogram

Sinus rhythm with normal heart rate (70 bpm), normal atrioventricular and intraventricular conduction, no ST-segment abnormalities or signs of LVH (aVL 0.3 mV; Sokolow–Lyon: 2.5 mV; Cornell voltage 0.7 mV; Cornell product 67.9 mV*ms) (Fig. 5.2).

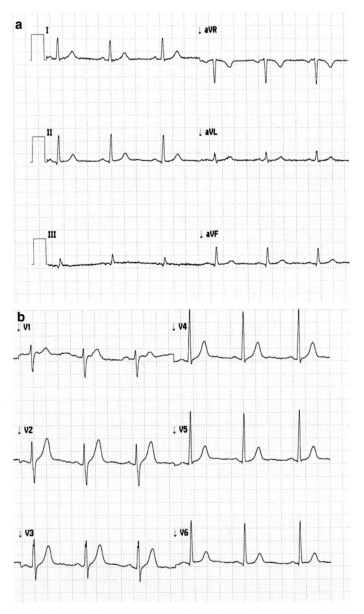

FIGURE 5.2 12-lead electrocardiogram at first visit: sinus rhythm with normal heart rate (70 bpm), normal atrioventricular and intraventricular conduction, no ST-segment abnormalities or signs of LVH. Peripheral (**a**) and precordial (**b**) leads

Echocardiogram with Doppler Ultrasound

Normal LV geometry (LV mass indexed 88 g/m^2; relative wall thickness: 0.37) with normal chamber dimension (LV end-diastolic diameter 47 mm) (Fig. 5.3a), normal LV relaxation (E/A ratio 2.1) at conventional Doppler evaluation and normal ejection fraction (LV ejection fraction 67 %, LV fractional shortening 37 %). Normal dimensions of aortic root and left atrium. Right ventricle with normal dimension and function. Pericardium without relevant abnormalities.

Mitral (+) regurgitation at Doppler ultrasound examination.

Current Treatment

Lisinopril 10 mg h 8:00; nebivolol/HCTZ 5/25 mg h 12:00; lacidipine 6 mg h 20:00; aspirin 100 mg h 12:00; rosuvastatin 5 mg h 22:00

Diagnosis

Essential (stage 2) hypertension with unsatisfactory BP control on combination therapy. No evidence hypertension-related cardiac and renal organ damage. One additional modifiable cardiovascular risk factors, i.e. hypercholesterolaemia. No other relevant clinical conditions

Which is the global cardiovascular risk profile in this patient?

Possible answers are:

1. Low
2. Medium
3. High
4. Very high

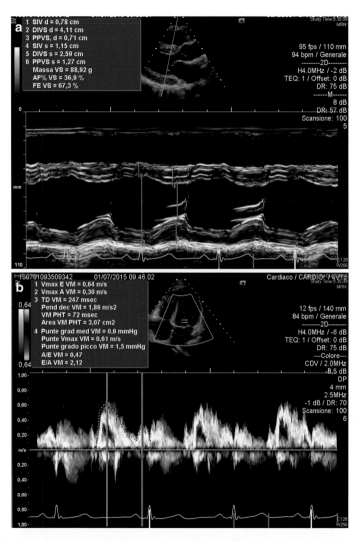

FIGURE 5.3 Echocardiogram with Doppler ultrasound at first visit: normal LV geometry with normal chamber dimension (**a**), normal LV relaxation at conventional Doppler evaluation (**b**) and normal ejection fraction. Normal dimensions of aortic root and left atrium. Right ventricle with normal dimension and function. Pericardium without relevant abnormalities. Mitral (+) regurgitation at Doppler ultrasound examination

Global Cardiovascular Risk Stratification

According to 2013 ESH/ESC global cardiovascular risk stratification [1], this patient has moderate to high cardiovascular risk.

> **Which is the best therapeutic option in this patient?**
> Possible answers are:
>
> 1. Add another drug class (e.g. loop diuretic).
> 2. Add another drug class (e.g. antialdosterone agent).
> 3. Titrate current therapy and switch to long-lasting agents.
> 4. Switch from ACE inhibitor to angiotensin receptor blocker.
> 5. Switch from ACE inhibitor to direct renin inhibitor.

Treatment Evaluation

- Stop lisinopril 10 mg and lacidipine 6 mg.
- Start fixed combination with perindopril/amlodipine 5/5 mg h 20:00.
- Maintain nebivolol/HCTZ 5/25 mg h 8:00, aspirin 100 mg h 12:00, rosuvastatin 5 mg h 22:00.

Prescriptions

- Periodical BP evaluation at home according to recommendations from guidelines
- Blood tests for lipid parameters, including total, LDL, HDL cholesterol and triglycerides
- Carotid Doppler ultrasound examination to exclude the presence of vascular organ damage

5.2   Follow-Up (Visit 1) at 6 Weeks

At follow-up visit, the patient is in good clinical condition. She reported good adherence to prescribed medications without adverse reactions or drug-related side effects.

Physical Examination

- Resting pulse: regular rhythm with normal heart rate (71 beats/min)
- Other clinical parameters substantially unchanged

Blood Pressure Profile

- Home BP (average): 145/95 mmHg
- Sitting BP: 143/96 mmHg (left arm)
- Standing BP: 145/98 mmHg at 1 min

Current Treatment

Nebivolol/HCTZ 5/25 mg h 8:00; perindopril/amlodipine 5/5 mg h 20:00; aspirin 100 mg h 12:00; rosuvastatin 5 mg h 22:00

Vascular Ultrasound

Carotid: intima–media thickness at both carotid levels (right: 1.0 mm; left: 1.0 mm) with evidence of fibro-calcific atherosclerotic plaque, located at right carotid bifurcation and internal carotid artery (Fig. 5.4a), resulting in 50 % stenosis of the vessel lumen (Fig. 5.4b)

Renal: intima–media thickness at both renal arteries without evidence of atherosclerotic plaques. Normal Doppler evaluation at both right and left renal arteries (main vessels and intraparenchymal arteries). Normal dimension and structure of the abdominal aorta

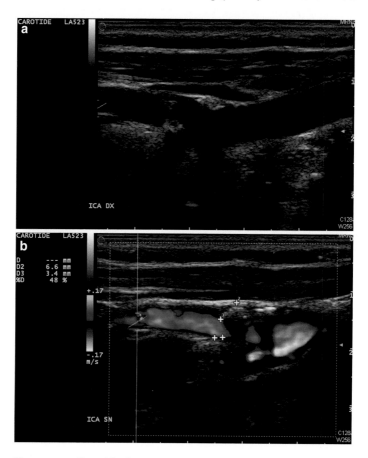

FIGURE 5.4 Carotid ultrasound at follow-up visit after 6 weeks: intima–media thickness at both carotid levels (right: 1.0 mm; left: 1.0 mm) with evidence of fibro-calcific atherosclerotic plaque, located at the right carotid bifurcation and internal carotid artery (**a**), resulting in 50 % stenosis of the vessel lumen (**b**)

Haematological Profile

- Fasting lipids: total cholesterol (TOT-C), 192 mg/dl; low-density lipoprotein cholesterol (LDL-C), 121 mg/dl; high-density lipoprotein cholesterol (HDL-C), 40 mg/dl; triglycerides (TG) 156 mg/dl

Diagnosis

Essential (stage 1) hypertension with improved BP control on combination therapy without achieving the recommended BP targets. Vascular organ damage (carotid atherosclerosis). Hypercholesterolaemia. No additional cardiovascular risk factors, markers or hypertension-related organ damage nor associated clinical conditions

Which is the global cardiovascular risk profile in this patient?

Possible answers are:

1. Low
2. Medium
3. High
4. Very high

Global Cardiovascular Risk Stratification

The ultrasound evidence of vascular organ damage (carotid atherosclerosis) is able to modify the individual global cardiovascular risk profile. On the basis of this assessment, this patient has moved from moderate to high to high cardiovascular risk, according to 2013 ESH/ESC global cardiovascular risk stratification [1]. This would lead to an increased 10-year risk of developing cardiovascular disease (morbidity and mortality).

Which is the best therapeutic option in this patient?

Possible answers are:

1. Add another drug class (e.g. loop diuretic).
2. Add another drug class (e.g. antialdosterone agent).
3. Titrate current therapy.
4. Switch from ACE inhibitor to angiotensin receptor blocker.
5. Switch from CE inhibitor to direct renin inhibitor.

Treatment Evaluation

- Titrate perindopril/amlodipine from 5/5 mg to 10/5 mg h 20:00.
- Titrate rosuvastatin from 5 to 20 mg.
- Maintain nebivolol/HCTZ 5/25 mg h 8:00 and aspirin 100 mg h 12:00.

Prescriptions

- Periodical BP evaluation at home according to recommendations from current guidelines
- Blood tests for lipid parameters, including total, LDL, HDL cholesterol and triglycerides, liver and muscular functions

5.3   Follow-Up (Visit 2) at 3 Months

At follow-up visit, the patient is in good clinical condition. She reported good adherence to prescribed medications without adverse reactions or drug-related side effects.

Physical Examination

- Resting pulse: regular rhythm with 72 beats/min
- Other parameters substantially unchanged

Blood Pressure Profile

- Home BP (average): 140/90 mmHg
- Sitting BP: 141/92 mmHg (left arm)
- Standing BP: 142/95 mmHg at 1 min

Current Treatment

Nebivolol/HCTZ 5/25 mg h 8:00; perindopril/amlodipine 10/5 mg h 20:00; aspirin 100 mg h 12:00; rosuvastatin 20 mg h 22:00

Haematological Profile

- Fasting lipids: total cholesterol (TOT-C), 146 mg/dl; low-density lipoprotein cholesterol (LDL-C), 83 mg/dl; high-density lipoprotein cholesterol (HDL-C), 44 mg/dl; triglycerides (TG) 98 mg/dl

Which is the best therapeutic option in this patient?
Possible answers are:

1. Add another drug class (e.g. loop diuretic).
2. Add another drug class (e.g. antialdosterone agent).
3. Titrate current therapy.
4. Switch from ACE inhibitor to angiotensin receptor blocker.
5. Switch from CE inhibitor to direct renin inhibitor.

Treatment Evaluation

- Titrate perindopril/amlodipine from 10/5 mg to 10/10 mg h 20:00.
- Maintain nebivolol/HCTZ 5/25 mg h 8:00, aspirin 100 mg h 12:00, and rosuvastatin 20 mg h 22:00.

Prescriptions

- Periodical BP evaluation at home according to recommendations from current guidelines.
- Repeat the 24-h ambulatory BP monitoring to test sustained and effective antihypertensive efficacy of prescribed medications.

5.4   Follow-Up (Visit 2) at 1 Year

At follow-up visit, the patient is in good clinical condition. She also reported good adherence to prescribed medications with no adverse reactions or relevant drug-related side effects.

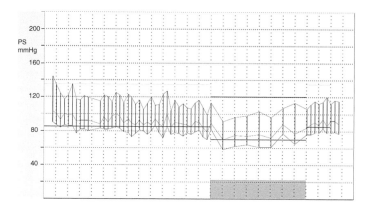

FIGURE 5.5 24-h ambulatory blood pressure profile at follow-up visit after 1 year

Physical Examination

- Resting pulse: regular rhythm with 72 beats/min
- Other parameters substantially unchanged

Blood Pressure Profile

- Home BP (average): 120/80 mmHg
- Sitting BP: 131/81 mmHg (left arm)
- Standing BP: 136/83 mmHg at 1 min
- 24-h BP: 115/78 mmHg; HR: 78 bpm
- Daytime BP: 117/80 mmHg; HR: 80 bpm
- Night-time BP: 102/66 mmHg; HR: 64 bpm

The 24-h ambulatory blood pressure profile is illustrated in Fig. 5.5.

Current Treatment

- Nebivolol/HCTZ 5/25 mg h 8:00, perindopril/amlodipine from 10/10 mg h 20:00, aspirin 100 mg h 12:00, rosuvastatin from 5 to 20 mg

Treatment Evaluation

No changes for current pharmacological therapy

Prescriptions

- Periodical BP evaluation at home according to recommendations from current guidelines
- Blood tests for lipid parameters, including total, LDL, HDL cholesterol and triglycerides, liver and muscular functions

---

Which is the most useful diagnostic test to repeat during the follow-up in this patient?

Possible answers are:

1. Electrocardiogram
2. Echocardiogram
3. Vascular Doppler ultrasound
4. Evaluation of renal parameters (e.g. creatininemia, eGFR, ClCr, UACR)
5. 24-h ambulatory BP monitoring

5.5   Discussion

Essential hypertension has been associated to an increased risk of development and progression of vascular organ damage, independently by the concomitant presence of diabetes or other metabolic abnormalities. Hypertension-related atherosclerosis can be observed at different levels of the arterial vasculature, including coronary, aortic, carotid, cerebral, renal and peripheral arteries. Whatever the arterial segment affected, once established, the presence of atherosclerosis has been related to an increased risk of coronary events, myocardial infarction, ischemic stroke, renal failure, peripheral *claudication* and ischaemia. Also, these abnormalities have been observed in both large and small vessels of hypertensive patients, thus inducing an increased risk of macrovascular or microvascular complications, respectively.

For these reasons, systematic assessment of structural and functional abnormalities of the vasculature in all hypertensive patients has been recently reaffirmed and promoted by the 2013 European Society of Hypertension (ESH)/European Society of Cardiology (ESC) guidelines on the clinical management of hypertension [1], in order to properly identify and treat those hypertensive patients at high cardiovascular risk.

In this view, the presence of atherosclerotic plaques can be assessed with various diagnostic tests, depending on the arterial segment to be evaluated, although with different levels of sensitivity and specificity. In a setting clinical practice, the most commonly used test is represented by the Doppler ultrasound examination of the carotid arteries, followed by the Doppler analysis of the abdominal aorta and renal and lower limb arteries. With these tests, several information on the vascular structure and function can be obtained in a noninvasive, simply and effective way.

Beyond the presence or absence of atherosclerotic plaques, automatic or semiautomatic assessment of the intima–media thickness as well as quantification of the blood flow velocity through the artery can be achieved. It should be noted, however, that although current guidelines recognised only the presence of atherosclerotic plaques (with or without haemodynamic effects) as marker of vascular organ damage [1], the presence of either intima–media thickness or increased blood flow velocity can be viewed as an early marker of vascular damage. These data may be of potential clinical useful for the referring physicians, in order to early identify those hypertensive patients who may develop established vascular organ damage during an early, asymptomatic stage of the disease, thus implementing the most appropriate pharmacological therapy to prevent the development and reduce the progression of atherosclerotic lesions.

In this clinical case, some aspects deserve a comment. First of all, Doppler ultrasound evaluation of vascular organ damage should be always performed in all hypertensive patients, if available, especially in those with diabetes, metabolic abnormalities or lipid disorders, in order to evaluate vascular structure and function. The search for vascular organ damage can be performed at carotid level in a first diagnostic step and then implemented with the analysis at either abdominal, renal or peripheral level, according to the presence of specific signs or symptoms of renal impairment or peripheral artery disease.

In this latter regard, it should be also noted, however, that the presence of atherosclerosis at one vessel segment leads to high probability of having other segments affected by atherosclerotic lesions. This may have relatively limited effect on global cardiovascular risk stratification (i.e. the individual global cardiovascular risk profile remains high for the presence of vascular organ damage, independently by the absolute number of affected segments or degree of vascular stenosis) but relevant consequences for the clinical management of these hypertensive patients, who need a more integrated and intensive pharmacological strategy, in order to reduce the risk of major cardiovascular complications.

In this patient, the Doppler evidence of carotid atherosclerosis has two major consequences. From the patient's point of view, she was definitely motivated to assume the prescribed pharmacological therapy, which included high dose of BP-lowering and lipid-lowering drugs. From the doctor's point of view, this evidence was able to modify her global cardiovascular risk profile from moderate to high, which had important clinical consequences. Indeed, the presence of vascular organ damage may help physicians in choosing among different antihypertensive drug classes and tailoring the most effective antihypertensive therapy at appropriate dosages and/or combination, according to compelling indications from current hypertension guidelines [1]. For example, the therapeutic choice for this patient was oriented on a fixed combination therapy based on the beta-blocker and thiazide diuretic in the morning and a fixed combination therapy with the ACE inhibitor perindopril and the dihydropyridinine calcium-channel blocker amlodipine in the evening. With the facilities of having multiple drug principles in two separate pills, this strategy has demonstrated beneficial effects on cardiovascular morbidity and mortality in hypertensive patients with vascular organ [2, 3].

In the preliminary evaluation of the patient, the main goal of the therapeutic strategy was focused on the BP reduction, since there was no evidence of uncontrolled additional cardiovascular risk factors or markers of organ damage. In a subsequent step, the discovery of vascular organ damage induced an up-titration of both antihypertensive and lipid-lowering therapies throughout the adoption of antihypertensive drug classes and high-dose statin therapy with proven benefits on regression of vascular atherosclerosis, beyond BP- and lipid-lowering efficacy.

During the follow-up evaluation of this hypertensive patient with vascular organ damage, repeated Doppler ultrasound evaluations of atherosclerotic plaques may provide indirect evidence of the therapeutic effectiveness of antihypertensive therapy, by demonstrating the regression of vascular atherosclerosis, a phenomenon that has been associated to a reduced risk of cardiovascular and cerebrovascular complications.

Take-Home Messages
- The presence of vascular organ damage (namely, atherosclerotic plaque) increases the risk of developing major cardiovascular and cerebrovascular complications in hypertension.
- The regression of atherosclerotic plaque, beyond the achievement of effective BP control, has been associated with improved cardiovascular prognosis.
- All hypertensive patients should undergo Doppler ultrasound examination, in order to assess the presence

atherosclerotic plaque, particularly in the presence of diabetes, metabolic abnormalities and lipid disorders.

- The most commonly used test applied in a setting of clinical practice is represented by the examination of vascular structure and function at carotid level.
- Other arterial segment (cerebral, coronary, abdominal, renal and peripheral arteries) can be evaluated with specific diagnostic tests, the use of which should be limited in the presence of specific signs and/or symptoms of vascular damage.
- In view of the large diffusion, relatively high reproducibility and non-invasive approach, this exam can be repeated during the follow-up, to evaluate potential regression of atherosclerosis at various levels.

References

1. Mancia G, Fagard R, Narkiewicz K, Redon J, Zanchetti A, Bohm M, et al. 2013 ESH/ESC Guidelines for the management of arterial hypertension: the Task Force for the management of arterial hypertension of the European Society of Hypertension (ESH) and of the European Society of Cardiology (ESC). J Hypertens. 2013;31(7):1281–357.
2. Dahlof B, Sever PS, Poulter NR, Wedel H, Beevers DG, Caulfield M, et al. Prevention of cardiovascular events with an antihypertensive regimen of amlodipine adding perindopril as required versus atenolol adding bendroflumethiazide as required, in the Anglo-Scandinavian Cardiac Outcomes Trial-Blood Pressure Lowering Arm (ASCOT-BPLA): a multicentre randomised controlled trial. Lancet. 2005;366(9489):895–906.
3. Sever PS, Dahlof B, Poulter NR, Wedel H, Beevers G, Caulfield M, et al. Prevention of coronary and stroke events with atorvastatin in hypertensive patients who have average or lower-than-average cholesterol concentrations, in the Anglo-Scandinavian Cardiac Outcomes Trial – Lipid Lowering Arm (ASCOT-LLA): a multicentre randomised controlled trial. Drugs. 2004;64 Suppl 2:43–60.

Clinical Case 6
Patient with Essential Hypertension and High Pulse Pressure

6.1 Clinical Case Presentation

An 81-year-old, Caucasian male, former CEO of chemical company, presented to the Outpatient Clinic for uncontrolled systolic hypertension.

He has history of essential, isolated systolic hypertension by more than 20 years, treated with a combination therapy based on ACE inhibitor (ramipril 10 mg), diuretic (furosemide 25 mg), beta-blocker (bisoprolol 2.5 mg) and alpha-blocker (doxazosin 4 mg).

About 10 years ago, he was switched from ACE inhibitor to angiotensin receptor blocker (losartan 100 mg) for uncontrolled BP levels and evidence of cardiac organ damage (namely, LV hypertrophy). He was also stropped from calcium-channel blocker (nifedipine slow release 30 mg), due to lower limb oedema, palpitations and persistently uncontrolled BP levels, and then moved to alpha-blocker (doxazosin 4 mg) without relevant side effects, although with limited improvement of blood pressure (BP) control.

By about 6 months, he reported markedly uncontrolled BP levels measured at home, particularly for the systolic and during the early morning. Thus, his referring physician prescribed to doubling the dosage of doxazosin 4 mg twice daily in

G. Tocci, *Hypertension and Organ Damage: A Case-Based Guide to Management*, Practical Case Studies in Hypertension Management, DOI 10.1007/978-3-319-25097-7_6,
© Springer International Publishing Switzerland 2016

addition to current pharmacological therapy, albeit with persistently high systolic BP levels at home. He also described symptomatic hypotension.

Family History

He has paternal history of hypertension and stroke and maternal history of hypertension and diabetes. He also has one brother and one sister with hypertension and one sister with coronary artery disease.

Clinical History

He was a previous smoker (about 10–20 cigarettes daily) for more than 30 years until the age of 60 years. He also has two additional modifiable cardiovascular risk factors, including overweight (visceral obesity) and hypercholesterolaemia treated with simvastatin 20 mg. There were no further cardio-vascular risk factors, associated clinical conditions or non-cardiovascular diseases.

He reported regular physical activity (1-h aerobic section 2–3 times per week). For this reason, his referring physician prescribed electrocardiogram and blood tests annually, as well as echocardiogram and exercise stress test every 2–3 years in the absence of specific signs or symptoms of effort dyspnoea or angina.

Physical Examination

- Weight: 86 kg
- Height: 178 cm
- Body mass index (BMI): 27.1 kg/m^2
- Waist circumference: 114 cm
- Respiration: normal
- Heart sounds: S1–S2 regular, normal, no murmurs

- Resting pulse: regular rhythm with normal heart rate (62 beats/min)
- Carotid arteries: no murmurs
- Femoral and foot arteries: palpable

Haematological Profile

- Haemoglobin: 14.3 g/dL
- Haematocrit: 50.2 %
- Fasting plasma glucose: 76 mg/dL
- Fasting lipids: total cholesterol (TOT-C), 168 mg/dl; low-density lipoprotein cholesterol (LDL-C), 100 mg/dl; high-density lipoprotein cholesterol (HDL-C), 41 mg/dl; triglycerides (TG) 138 mg/dl
- Electrolytes: sodium, 142 mEq/L; potassium, 4.0 mEq/L
- Serum uric acid: 5.1 mg/dL
- Renal function: urea, 26 mg/dl; creatinine, 1.0 mg/dL; creatinine clearance (Cockcroft–Gault), 71 ml/min; estimated glomerular filtration rate (eGFR) (MDRD), 80 mL/min/1.73 m^2
- Urine analysis (dipstick): proteinuria 10 mg/dl
- Normal liver function tests
- Normal thyroid function tests

Blood Pressure Profile

- Home BP (average): 150–160/70 mmHg
- Sitting BP: 168/75 mmHg (right arm); 166/78 mmHg (left arm)
- Standing BP: 160/78 mmHg at 1 min
- 24-h BP: 150/79 mmHg; HR: 81 bpm
- Daytime BP: 146/78 mmHg; HR: 83 bpm
- Night-time BP: 165/85 mmHg; HR: 72 bpm

The 24-h ambulatory blood pressure profile is illustrated in Fig. 6.1.

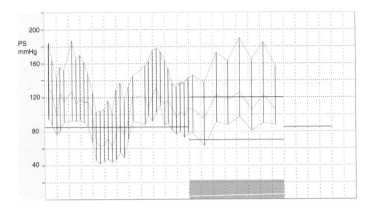

FIGURE 6.1 24-h ambulatory blood pressure profile at first visit

12-Lead Electrocardiogram

Sinus rhythm with normal heart rate (59 bpm), normal atrio-ventricular and intraventricular conduction, ST-segment abnormalities (reverse T waves) with signs of LVH (aVL 0.7 mV; Sokolow–Lyon, 3.8 mV; Cornell voltage 0.8 mV; Cornel product 81 mV*ms) (Fig. 6.2).

Vascular Ultrasound

Carotid: intima–media thickness at both carotid levels (right: 1.1 mm, bilaterally) with evidence of fibro-calcific atherosclerotic plaque at carotid bifurcation and internal carotid artery without haemodynamic effects (Fig. 6.3)

Renal: intima–media thickness at both renal arteries without evidence of atherosclerotic plaques. Normal Doppler examination at both right and left arteries. Normal dimension and structure of the abdominal aorta

Echocardiogram

Eccentric LV hypertrophy (LV mass indexed 124 g/m²; relative wall thickness: 0.41) with high-normal chamber dimension (LV end-diastolic diameter 56 mm) (Fig. 6.4a), impaired LV

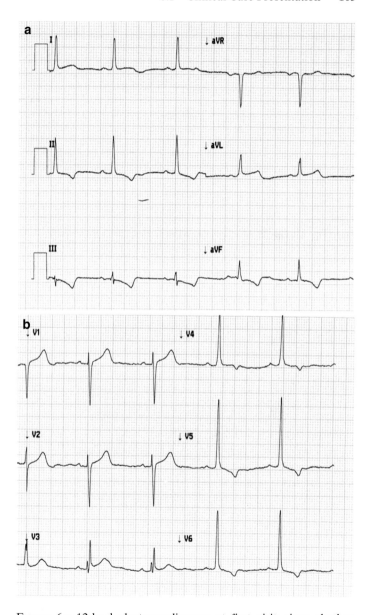

FIGURE 6.2 12-lead electrocardiogram at first visit: sinus rhythm with normal heart rate (59 bpm), normal atrioventricular and intra-ventricular conduction, ST-segment abnormalities (reverse T waves) with signs of LVH. Peripheral (**a**) and precordial (**b**) leads

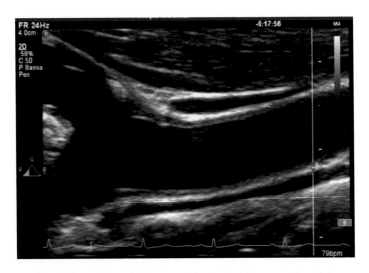

FIGURE 6.3 Carotid ultrasound at first visit: intima–media thickness at both carotid levels (right: 1.1 mm, bilaterally) with evidence of fibro-calcific atherosclerotic plaque at carotid bifurcation and internal carotid artery without haemodynamic effects

relaxation (E/A ratio 1.1) at conventional (Fig. 6.4b) Doppler evaluations and normal ejection fraction (LV ejection fraction 77 %, LV fractional shortening 46 %). Normal dimension of aortic root. High-normal dimension of left atrium (diameter 40 mm, area 26 cm^2). Right ventricle with normal dimension and function. Mild pericardial effusion without haemodynamic effects

Mitral (+) and tricuspid (+) regurgitations at Doppler ultrasound examination

Current Treatment

Losartan 100 mg h 8:00; furosemide 25 mg h 8:00; bisoprolol 2.5 mg h 8:00; aspirin 100 mg; doxazosin 4 mg h 22:00; simvastatin 20 mg h 22:00

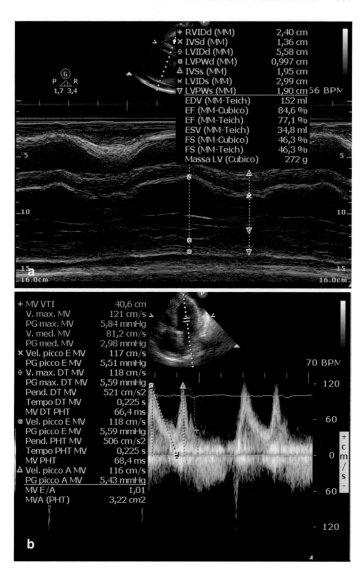

FIGURE 6.4 Echocardiogram at first visit: eccentric LV hypertrophy with high-normal chamber dimension (**a**), impaired LV relaxation at conventional (**b**) Doppler evaluations and normal ejection fraction. Normal dimension of aortic root. High-normal dimension of left atrium. Right ventricle with normal dimension and function. Mild pericardial effusion without haemodynamic effects. Mitral (+) and tricuspid (+) regurgitations at Doppler ultrasound examination

Diagnosis

Essential (stage 2) hypertension and isolated systolic hypertension with unsatisfactory BP control on combination therapy. High pulse pressure. Additional modifiable cardiovascular risk factors, including visceral obesity and hypercholesterolaemia. Evidence of hypertension-related cardiac and vascular organ damage. No associated clinical conditions.

Which is the global cardiovascular risk profile in this patient?

Possible answers are:

1. Low
2. Medium
3. High
4. Very high

Global Cardiovascular Risk Stratification

According to 2013 ESH/ESC global cardiovascular risk stratification [1], this patient has high cardiovascular risk.

Which is the best therapeutic option in this patient?

Possible answers are:

1. Add another drug class (e.g. dihydropyridinic calcium antagonist).
2. Add another drug class (e.g. antialdosterone agent).
3. Add another drug class (e.g. direct renin inhibitor).
4. Switch to long-lasting ACE inhibitor.
5. Switch to long-lasting angiotensin receptor blocker.

Treatment Evaluation

- Stop losartan 100 mg and furosemide 25 mg.
- Start fixed combination therapy with olmesartan/hydro-chlorothiazide 20/25 mg h 8:00.
- Maintain bisoprolol 2.5 mg h 8:00, aspirin 100 mg, doxazo-sin 4 mg h 22:00, simvastatin 20 mg h 22:00.

Prescriptions

- Periodical BP evaluation at home according to recommendations from guidelines
- Moderate physical activity to reduced abdominal overweight
- Blood and urinary tests for renal parameters, including serum creatinine, urea estimated glomerular filtration rate and creatinine clearance, and urinary albumin/creatinine ratio on morning urine sample

6.2   Follow-Up (Visit 1) at 6 Weeks

At follow-up visit, the patient is in good clinical condition. He reported good adherence to prescribed medications without adverse reactions or drug-related side effects.

Physical Examination

- Waist circumference: 112 cm
- Resting pulse: regular rhythm with normal heart rate (66 beats/min)
- Other clinical parameters substantially unchanged

Blood Pressure Profile

- Home BP (average): 150/70 mmHg (early morning)
- Sitting BP: 156/76 mmHg (left arm)
- Standing BP: 158/74 mmHg at 1 min

Current Treatment

Olmesartan/hydrochlorothiazide 20/25 mg h 8:00; bisoprolol 2.5 mg h 8:00; doxazosin 4 mg h 22:00; aspirin 100 mg h 12:00; simvastatin 20 mg h 22:00

Haematological Profile

- Electrolytes: sodium, 143 mEq/L; potassium, 4.2 mEq/L
- Renal function: urea, 24 mg/dl; creatinine, 1.0 mg/dL; creatinine clearance (Cockcroft–Gault), 71 ml/min; estimated glomerular filtration rate (eGFR) (MDRD), 81 mL/min/1.73 m^2
- Urinary albumin/creatinine ratio (morning urine sample): 16 mg/g

Diagnosis

Essential (stage 2) hypertension and isolated systolic hypertension with improved BP control on combination therapy, without achieving the recommended BP targets. High pulse pressure. Additional modifiable cardiovascular risk factors, including visceral obesity and hypercholesterolaemia. Evidence of hypertension-related cardiac and vascular organ damage. No associated clinical conditions

Which is the global cardiovascular risk profile in this patient?

Possible answers are:

1. Low
2. Medium
3. High
4. Very high

Global Cardiovascular Risk Stratification

Although BP levels have been reduced and renal parameters remained substantially unchanged, this patient has persistently high cardiovascular risk, according to 2013 ESH/ESC global cardiovascular risk stratification [1], due to the presence of high pulse pressure and markers of cardiac and vascular organ damage.

Which is the best therapeutic option in this patient?
Possible answers are:

1. Add another drug class (e.g. dihydropyridinic calcium antagonist).
2. Add another drug class (e.g. antialdosterone agent).
3. Add another drug class (e.g. direct renin inhibitor).
4. Switch to long-lasting ACE inhibitor.
5. Titrate the dosage of current therapy.

Treatment Evaluation

- Titrate the dosage of olmesartan/hydrochlorothiazide from 20/25 mg to 40/25 mg h 8:00.
- Maintain bisoprolol 2.5 mg h 8:00, aspirin 100 mg, doxazosin 4 mg h 22:00 and simvastatin 20 mg h 22:00.

Prescriptions

- Periodical BP evaluation at home according to recommendations from current guidelines
- Moderate physical activity to reduced abdominal overweight
- Blood and urinary tests for renal parameters, including serum creatinine, urea estimated glomerular filtration rate and creatinine clearance, and urinary dipstick on morning urine sample.

6.3   Follow-Up (Visit 2) at 3 Months

At follow-up visit, the patient is in good clinical condition. He maintained regular physical activity two to three times per week with benefits (further weight loss and good exercise tolerance). He also reported good adherence to prescribed medications. However, he also described several episodes of symptomatic hypotension, particularly at bedtime.

Physical Examination

- Waist circumference: 111 cm
- Resting pulse: regular rhythm with 64 beats/min
- Other parameters substantially unchanged

Blood Pressure Profile

- Home BP (average): 135/70 mmHg (early morning)
- Sitting BP: 139/86 mmHg (left arm)
- Standing BP: 139/85 mmHg at 1 min

Current Treatment

Olmesartan/hydrochlorothiazide 40/25 mg h 8:00; bisoprolol 2.5 mg h 8:00; doxazosin 4 mg h 22:00; simvastatin 20 mg h 22:00

Which is the best therapeutic option in this patient?

Potential answers are:

1. Stop beta-blocker.
2. Stop alpha-blocker.
3. Stop thiazide diuretic.
4. Stop combination therapy with angiotensin receptor blocker and thiazide diuretic.
5. Reduce the dosage of current therapy.

Treatment Evaluation

- Stop doxazosin 4 mg.
- Olmesartan/hydrochlorothiazide 20/25 mg h 8:00; bisoprolol 2.5 mg h 8:00; aspirin 100 mg h 12:00; simvastatin 20 mg h 22:00.

Prescriptions

- Periodical BP evaluation at home according to recommendations from current guidelines.
- Blood and urinary tests for renal parameters, including serum creatinine, urea estimated glomerular filtration rate and creatinine clearance, and urinary albumin/creatinine ratio on morning urine sample.
- Repeat the 24-h ambulatory BP monitoring to test sustained and effective antihypertensive efficacy of prescribed medications.
- Repeat echocardiogram to evaluate LV mass and hypertrophy, systolic and diastolic function as well as pericardial effusion.

6.4   Follow-Up (Visit 2) at 1 Year

At follow-up visit, the patient is in good clinical condition. He reported good adherence to prescribed medications with no adverse reactions or relevant drug-related side effects.

Physical Examination

- Weight: 83 kg
- Waist circumference: 110 cm
- Resting pulse: regular rhythm with 62 beats/min
- Other parameters substantially unchanged

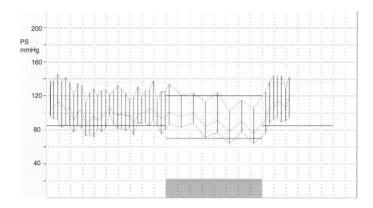

FIGURE 6.5 24-h ambulatory blood pressure profile at follow-up visit after 1 year

Blood Pressure Profile

- Home BP (average): 135/70 mmHg (early morning)
- Sitting BP: 138/84 mmHg (left arm)
- Standing BP: 137/86 mmHg at 1 min
- 24-h BP: 127/84 mmHg; HR: 79 bpm
- Daytime BP: 129/85 mmHg; HR: 80 bpm
- Night-time BP: 117/70 mmHg; HR: 70 bpm

The 24-h ambulatory blood pressure profile is illustrated in Fig. 6.5.

Haematological Profile

- Renal function: urea, 20 mg/dl; creatinine, 1.1 mg/dL; creatinine clearance (Cockcroft–Gault), 63 ml/min; estimated glomerular filtration rate (eGFR) (MDRD), 76 mL/min/1.73 m^2
- Urine analysis (dipstick): absence of proteinuria
- Urinary albumin/creatinine ratio (morning urine sample): 8 mg/g

Echocardiogram

Eccentric LV hypertrophy (LV mass indexed 120 g/m^2; relative wall thickness: 0.40) with high-normal chamber dimension (LV end-diastolic diameter 56 mm), impaired LV relaxation (E/A ratio 1.0) at conventional Doppler evaluations and normal ejection fraction (LV ejection fraction 75 %, LV fractional shortening 43 %). Normal dimension of aortic root. High-normal dimension of left atrium (diameter 39 mm, area 22 cm^2). Right ventricle with normal dimension and function. Pericardium without relevant abnormalities

Mitral (+) and tricuspid (+) regurgitations at Doppler ultrasound examination

Current Treatment

Olmesartan/hydrochlorothiazide 20/25 mg h 8:00; bisoprolol 2.5 mg h 8:00; aspirin 100 mg h 12:00; simvastatin 20 mg h 22:00

Treatment Evaluation

- No changes for current pharmacological therapy

Prescriptions

- Periodical BP evaluation at home according to recommendations from current guidelines
- Regular physical activity and low caloric intake

Which is the most useful diagnostic test to repeat during the follow-up in this patient?

Possible answers are:

1. Electrocardiogram
2. Echocardiogram
3. Vascular Doppler ultrasound
4. Evaluation of renal parameters (e.g. creatininaemia, eGFR, ClCr, UACR)
5. 24-h ambulatory BP monitoring

6.5   Discussion

Arterial hypertension, mostly isolated systolic hypertension, is a relatively frequent condition in elderly individuals, thus increasing the risk of developing major cardiovascular and cerebrovascular complications and heavily affecting prognosis of non-cardiovascular disease. Also, the need of assuming anti-hypertensive drugs should be carefully balanced with the potential effective of excessive BP reductions on cognitive function and, mostly, with the potential risk of multiple drug interactions with other concomitant therapies. For these reasons, as well as for the relatively limited evidence currently available in the very elderly population of hypertensive patients, the 2013 European Society of Hypertension (ESH)/ European Society of Cardiology (ESC) guidelines for the clinical management of hypertension [1] recommended that in fit elderly hypertensive patients aged less than 80 years the systolic BP levels be lowered to between 140 and 150 mmHg, if treatment is well tolerated. At the same time, in elderly hypertensive patients aged more than 80 years with an initial systolic BP more than 160 mmHg it is recommended to reduce systolic BP to between 150 and 140 mmHg, provided they are in good physical and mental conditions [1]. On the contrary, in frail elderly patients, it is recommended to leave decisions on antihypertensive therapy to the treating physician, and based on monitoring of the clinical effects of treatment [1].

In this clinical case some aspects deserve a comment. First of all, the elderly hypertensive patient was in good clinical condition without signs of cognitive decline or other relevant comorbidities. Also, he reported regular physical activity without signs or symptoms of cardiovascular or non-cardiovascular diseases. As discussed above, current European guidelines recommended for this patient to reduce systolic BP levels to target and even lower, if tolerated and not contraindicated.

This patient was previously treated with several antihypertensive drug classes or molecules, which induced drug-related adverse effects or side reactions. This is a common event in relatively long history of hypertensive disease, which may induce low adherence to prescribed medications from the patient point of view, and the use of several drug classes at relatively low dosages from the medical point of view. Both these actions can be related to the potential risk of having side effects, thus reducing the clinical efficacy of antihypertensive therapy.

Although current European guidelines recommended that all antihypertensive drug classes can be used in elderly hypertensive patients, calcium channel blockers and diuretics should be preferred. In this case, previous antihypertensive therapy with calcium channel blockers induced peripheral oedema and ACE inhibitors were stopped due to lack of antihypertensive efficacy. For these reasons, the subsequent switch from a relatively short-lasting (losartan) to a long-lasting (olmesartan) angiotensin receptor blocker and from a loop (furosemide) to a thiazide (hydrochlorothiazide) diuretic can be viewed in light of achieving a more effective, sustained and well-tolerated antihypertensive effect over the 24 h. Evidence are available and demonstrate the benefits obtained in terms of BP control from this antihypertensive strategy, which is also able to provide sustained antihypertensive efficacy [2–4].

During the follow-up evaluation of this elderly hypertensive patient with isolated systolic hypertension, the achievement of effective BP control without relevant drug-related side effects or adverse reactions allowed to stop concomitant therapies with limited antihypertensive efficacy or redundant effect. The optimization of antihypertensive strategy and the reduction of the pill burden have also demonstrated to positively affect adherence to prescribed medication in hypertension, through contributing to improve cardiovascular prognosis and the overall rate of BP control, even in high risk population of elderly hypertensive patients.

Take-Home Messages

- The presence of increased pulse pressure (namely isolated systolic hypertension) increases the risk of developing major cardiovascular complications in hypertension, mostly carotid atherosclerosis and ischemic stroke.
- In elderly hypertensive patients aged less than 80 years and having systolic BP more than 160 mmHg, it is recommended to reduce systolic BP levels to between 150 and 140 mmHg.
- In elderly hypertensive patients aged more than 80 years and with initial systolic BP more than 160 mmHg (as in this case), it is recommended to reduce systolic BP to between 150 and 140 mmHg provided they are in good physical and mental conditions.
- All hypertensive agents are recommended and can be used in the elderly, although diuretics and calcium antagonists may be preferred in isolated systolic hypertension.
- Recent evidence demonstrated that long-lasting antihypertensive drugs, particularly ACE inhibitors and angiotensin receptor blockers, may be effective and well-tolerated in elderly hypertensive patients aged more than 65 years.
- These drugs have demonstrated to reduce systolic BP levels to the recommended targets and to reduce cardiovascular morbidity and mortality, particularly ischemic stroke.

References

1. Mancia G, Fagard R, Narkiewicz K, Redon J, Zanchetti A, Bohm M, et al. 2013 ESH/ESC Guidelines for the management of arterial hypertension: the Task Force for the management of arterial hypertension of the European Society of Hypertension (ESH) and of the European Society of Cardiology (ESC). J Hypertens. 2013;31(7):1281–357.
2. Oparil S, Melino M, Lee J, Fernandez V, Heyrman R. Triple therapy with olmesartan medoxomil, amlodipine besylate, and hydrochlorothiazide in adult patients with hypertension: the TRINITY multicenter, randomized, double-blind, 12-week, parallel-group study. Clin Ther. 2010;32(7):1252–69.
3. Weir MR, Hsueh WA, Nesbitt SD, Littlejohn 3rd TJ, Graff A, Shojaee A, et al. A titrate-to-goal study of switching patients uncontrolled on antihypertensive monotherapy to fixed-dose combinations of amlodipine and olmesartan medoxomil +/– hydrochlorothiazide. J Clin Hypertens (Greenwich). 2011;13(6):404–12.
4. Malacco E, Omboni S, Volpe M, Auteri A, Zanchetti A. Antihypertensive efficacy and safety of olmesartan medoxomil and ramipril in elderly patients with mild to moderate essential hypertension: the ESPORT study. J Hypertens. 2010;28(11):2342–50.

Printed in the United States
By Bookmasters